Integrating Poverty and Gender into Health Programmes

A Sourcebook for Health Professionals

Module on HIV/AIDS

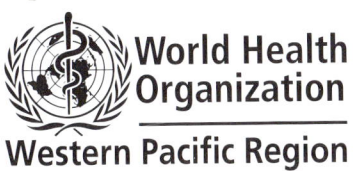

www.wpro.who.int

Photograph credits: cover, © 2005 Rick M. Reyes, Courtesy of Photoshare; pp. 1 © 2006 AYPagtan/CGN, Courtesy of Photoshare; pp. 3 © 2007 Jay Hubert, Courtesy of Photoshare; pp. 10 © 2004 Connelly La Mar, Courtesy of Photoshare; pp. 42 © 2006 Steven Nowakowski, Courtesy of Photoshare; pp. 71, 79 © 2005 Stéphane Janin, Courtesy of Photoshare; pp. 36 WHO/WPRO.

WHO Library Cataloguing in Publication Data

Integrating poverty and gender into health programmes: *a sourcebook for health professionals:* module on HIV/AIDS.

1. Acquired immunodeficiency syndrome. 2. HIV infections. 3. Poverty. 4. Gender. 5. Education, Professional. 6. Health programmes.

ISBN 13 978 92 9061 388 6 (NLM Classification: WA 30)

© World Health Organization 2008
All rights reserved.

The designations employed and the presentation of the material in this publication do not imply the expression of any opinion whatsoever on the part of the World Health Organization concerning the legal status of any country, territory, city or area or of its authorities, or concerning the delimitation of its frontiers or boundaries. Dotted lines on maps represent approximate border lines for which there may not yet be full agreement.

The mention of specific companies or of certain manufacturers' products does not imply that they are endorsed or recommended by the World Health Organization in preference to others of a similar nature that are not mentioned. Errors and omissions excepted, the names of proprietary products are distinguished by initial capital letters.

The World Health Organization does not warrant that the information contained in this publication is complete and correct and shall not be liable for any damages incurred as a result of its use.

Publications of the World Health Organization can be obtained from Marketing and Dissemination, World Health Organization, 20 Avenue Appia, 1211 Geneva 27, Switzerland (tel: +41 22 791 2476; fax: +41 22 791 4857; email: bookorders@who.int). Requests for permission to reproduce WHO publications, in part or in whole, or to translate them whether for sale or for noncommercial distribution should be addressed to Publications, at the above address (fax: +41 22 791 4806; email: permissions@who.int). For WHO Western Pacific Regional Publications, request for permission to reproduce should be addressed to Publications Office, World Health Organization, Regional Office for the Western Pacific, P.O. Box 2932, 1000, Manila, Philippines, Fax. No. (632) 521-1036, email: publications@wpro.who.int.

CONTENTS

ACKNOWLEDGEMENTS iv
ABBREVIATIONS v
PREFACE vi
INTRODUCTION 1

1. What is HIV/AIDS? 3
    WHO clinical staging system for HIV infection and disease 4
    The global burden of HIV/AIDS 5

2. What are the links between poverty, gender and HIV/AIDS? 10
    The links between poverty and HIV/AIDS 11
        The effect of poverty on HIV infection 13
        Progression from HIV to AIDS 20
        HIV/AIDS may cause or contribute to poverty 23
    The links between gender and HIV/AIDS 27
        Vulnerability of women and girls to HIV/AIDS 28
        Gender and the vulnerability of men and boys to HIV/AIDS 33

3. Why is it important for health professionals to address poverty and gender concerns in HIV/AIDS? 36
    Efficiency 37
    Equity 38
    Human rights 39

4. How can health professionals address poverty and gender concerns in HIV/AIDS? 42
    Policy level 43
        International policies 43
        National policies 45
    Financing 47
    Programme planning 48
    Prevention, treatment and care services 49
        Prevention 50
        Pro-poor and gender-sensitive voluntary HIV counselling and testing 61
        Treatment and care 63
        Monitoring and evaluation of poverty/equity and gender in HIV/AIDS 69
        Research 69

5. Facilitator's notes 71
    Expected learning outcomes 72
    Activity 1: Declarations on poverty and gender in HIV/AIDS 72

Activity 2: Influencing change...74

Activity 3: Case study problem-solving exercise..75

Activity 4: Planning poverty- and gender-sensitive HIV/AIDS programmes.....77

Workshop evaluation..78

6. Tools, resources and references...**79**

Tools..80

Resources..87

References...90

Endnotes..**110**

BOXES

Box 1:	Defining poverty..	11
Box 2:	Populations vulnerable to HIV/AIDS..	13
Box 3:	Experiences of women as family caregivers in Botswana...................	32
Box 4:	HIV, human rights and the Siracusa Principles...................................	39
Box 5:	HIV/AIDS and the accountability of states...	40
Box 6:	Global blueprint to stop and reverse the spread of HIV: MDG 6 and the UNGASS global targets for low- and middle-income countries.........................	44
Box 7:	AIDS and the Millennium Development Goals...................................	45
Box 8:	Mobilizing resources and providing opportunities for people infected with or affected by HIV/AIDS...	47
Box 9:	Prepayment scheme for health care for PLWH in Rwanda.................	48
Box 10:	Engaging the private sector in the response to AIDS: financing prevention and treatment for employees of a diamond mine in Botswana........................	49
Box 11:	Planning for the health sector with HIV in mind: the case of Sida.....	50
Box 12:	Integrating gender concerns into HIV/AIDS programming................	51
Box 13:	Developing effective HIV/AIDS prevention programmes...................	53
Box 14:	Promoting sexual health and citizenship through participatory methods to reduce the vulnerability of marginalized boys and young men in West Bengal, India........	54
Box 15:	Microbicides...	55
Box 16:	Family AIDS education and prevention in Uganda.............................	58
Box 17:	Women's health and HIV: a sex workers' project in Calcutta.............	59
Box 18:	Exploring sex and sexual relationships to support behavioural change among individuals and communities: the experience of Stepping Stones............	60
Box 19:	Making HIV counselling and testing work—some recommendations..	62
Box 20:	Reaching the poor in Rio de Janeiro..	65
Box 21:	Ensuring equal access for women and men..	67

Box 22:	Some international research efforts.	70
Box 23:	HIV/AIDS and gender- and poverty-sensitivity in health care services.	80
Box 24:	Checklist: Gender-sensitive PMTCT programmes.	80
Box 25:	Activities for poverty- and gender-sensitive VCT programmes	81
Box 27:	Expected achievements of an HIV/AIDS prevention programme	81
Box 28:	Twelve statements from the International Community of Women Living with HIV/AIDS.	82
Box 29:	Women and HIV/AIDS: The Barcelona Bill of Rights.	82
Box 30:	Evaluation of poverty- and gender-sensitive HIV/AIDS programmes.	83
Box 31:	HIV/AIDS and human rights	84
Box 32:	Mainstreaming gender equality and women's human rights: gender in one national AIDS action framework.	85
Box 33.	Examples of gender-sensitive HIV/AIDS indicators, with targets and information sources.	86

FIGURES

Figure 1:	Estimated number of people living with HIV (all ages), by WHO region, 2007.	6
Figure 2:	HIV prevalence among the general population in Cambodia, 1995–2006.	6
Figure 3:	Reported HIV infections by sex, Papua New Guinea, 1987–2006.	8
Figure 4:	The relationship between poverty and HIV/AIDS.	12
Figure 5:	Poverty increases the likelihood of HIV infection and AIDS.	14
Figure 6:	Proportion of women aged 15–49 years who know at least one way to avoid sexual transmission of HIV by income quintile, in Cambodia (2000), the Philippines (2003) and Viet Nam (2002).	15
Figure 7:	Proportion of men aged 15–54 years who know at least one way to avoid sexual transmission of HIV, by income quintile, in the Philippines.	15
Figure 8:	Proportion of girls aged 15–19 years who have at least one major misconception* about HIV/AIDS or had never heard of AIDS, 1999–2001.	19
Figure 9:	HIV/AIDS can induce and deepen poverty.	24
Figure 10:	Percentage of adults (15+) living with HIV who are female, 1990–2007.	28
Figure 11:	Comprehensive HIV/AIDS care and support.	52
Figure 12:	Women as a percentage of all adults receiving antiretroviral therapy in selected countries, actual verses expected percentages, 2005.	66

TABLES

Table 1:	WHO clinical staging of HIV/AIDS for adults and adolescents with confirmed HIV infection.	5
Table 2:	Global summary of the AIDS epidemic	5
Table 3:	HIV estimations for selected countries in the Western Pacific Region, 2005.	7

Table 4:	HIV and AIDS statistics and features in the Pacific	9
Table 5:	Estimated number of people with HIV/AIDS in China	9
Table 6:	Poverty, low education and risk-taking behaviour in Viet Nam	16
Table 7:	Estimated number of people receiving and needing antiretroviral therapy and the percentage coverage in low- and middle-income countries by region, June 2006	64

ACKNOWLEDGEMENTS

This module is one of a complete set entitled *Integrating Poverty and Gender into Health Programmes: A Sourcebook for Health Professionals*. It was prepared by a team comprising Sarah Coll-Black, Elizabeth Lindsay (consultants and principal writers), Anjana Bhushan (Technical Officer, Health in Development) and Kathleen Fritsch (Regional Adviser in Nursing) at the World Health Organization's Regional Office for the Western Pacific. Additional material was contributed by Ilia Smith. Breeda Hickey provided substantial supplementary inputs and also did preliminary editing of the module. Bernard Fabre-Teste, Gaik Gui Ong and Nguyen Thi Thanh Thuy provided thoughtful comments and helpful inputs. Rhonda Vandeworp did the final editing. Design and layout were done by Zando Escultura.

ABBREVIATIONS

AIDS	Acquired immunodeficiency syndrome
ARI	Acute respiratory infection
ART	Antiretroviral treatment or therapy
ARV	Antiretroviral
CEDAW	Convention on the Elimination of All Forms of Discrimination against Women
CRC	Convention of the Rights of the Child
DFID	Department for International Development of the United Kingdom
FBO	Faith-based organization
GDP	Gross domestic product
GFATM	Global Fund to Fight AIDS, Tuberculosis and Malaria
GHI	Global health initiative
GNI	Gross national income
GNP	Gross national product
HIV	Human immunodeficiency virus
ICW	International Community of Women
IDU	Injecting drug user
IEC	Information, education and communication
MCH	Maternal and child health
MDG	Millennium Development Goal
MTCT	Mother-to-child transmission
MSM	Men who have sex with men
NGO	Nongovernmental organization
NTP	National Tuberculosis Programme
OECD	Organisation for Economic Co-operation and Development
OI	Opportunistic infection
OVC	Orphans and vulnerable children
PEP	Post-exposure prophylaxis
PHC	Primary health care
PLWH	People living with HIV
PMTCT	Prevention of mother-to-child transmission
PRSP	Poverty Reduction Strategy Paper
RBM	Roll Back Malaria
RTI	Reproductive tract infection
SIDA	Swedish Agency for International Development Cooperation
SRH	Sexual and reproductive health
STI	Sexually transmitted infection
TB	Tuberculosis
UN	United Nations
UNAIDS	Joint United Nations Programme on HIV/AIDS
UNDP	United Nations Development Programme
UNGASS	United Nations General Assembly Special Session on HIV/AIDS
UNHCHR	United Nations High Commission for Human Rights
UNICEF	United Nations Children's Fund
UNIFEM	United Nations Development Fund for Women
VCT	Voluntary counselling and testing
WB	World Bank
WHO	World Health Organization

PREFACE

Over the past two to three decades, our understanding of poverty has broadened from a narrow focus on income and consumption to a multidimensional notion of education, health, social and political participation, personal security and freedom and environmental quality.[1] Thus, poverty encompasses not just low income, but lack of access to services, resources and skills; vulnerability; insecurity; and voicelessness and powerlessness. Multidimensional poverty is a determinant of health risks, health seeking behaviour, health care access and health outcomes.

As analyses of health outcomes become more refined, it is increasingly apparent that the impressive gains in health experienced over recent decades are unevenly distributed. Aggregate indicators, whether at the global, regional or national level, often tend to mask striking variations in health outcomes between men and women, rich and poor, both across and within countries.

An estimated 70% of the world's poor are women.[2] Similarly, in the Western Pacific Region, poverty often wears a woman's face. Indicators of human poverty, including health indicators, often reflect severe gender-based disparities. In this way, gender inequality is a significant determinant of health outcomes in the Region, with women and girls often at a severe societal disadvantage.

Although poverty and gender significantly influence health and socioeconomic development, health professionals are not always adequately prepared to address such issues in their work. This publication aims to improve the awareness, knowledge and skills of health professionals in the Region on poverty and gender concerns.

The modules that comprise this Sourcebook are intended for use in pre-service and in-service training of health professionals. This publication also is expected to be of use to health policy-makers and programme managers, either as a reference document or in conjunction with in-service training.

All modules in the series are linked, though each one can be used on a stand-alone basis if required. Two foundational modules establish the conceptual framework for the analysis of poverty and gender issues in health. Each of the other modules is intended for use in conjunction with these two foundational modules. The Sourcebook also contains a module on curricular integration to support health professional educational institutions integrate poverty and gender concerns into existing curricula.

All modules in the Sourcebook are designed for use through participatory learning methods that involve the learner, taking advantage of his or her experience and knowledge. Each module contains facilitators' notes and suggested exercises to assist in this process.

It is hoped that the Sourcebook will prove useful in bringing greater attention to poverty and gender concerns in the design, implementation and monitoring and evaluation of health policies, programmes and interventions.

Introduction

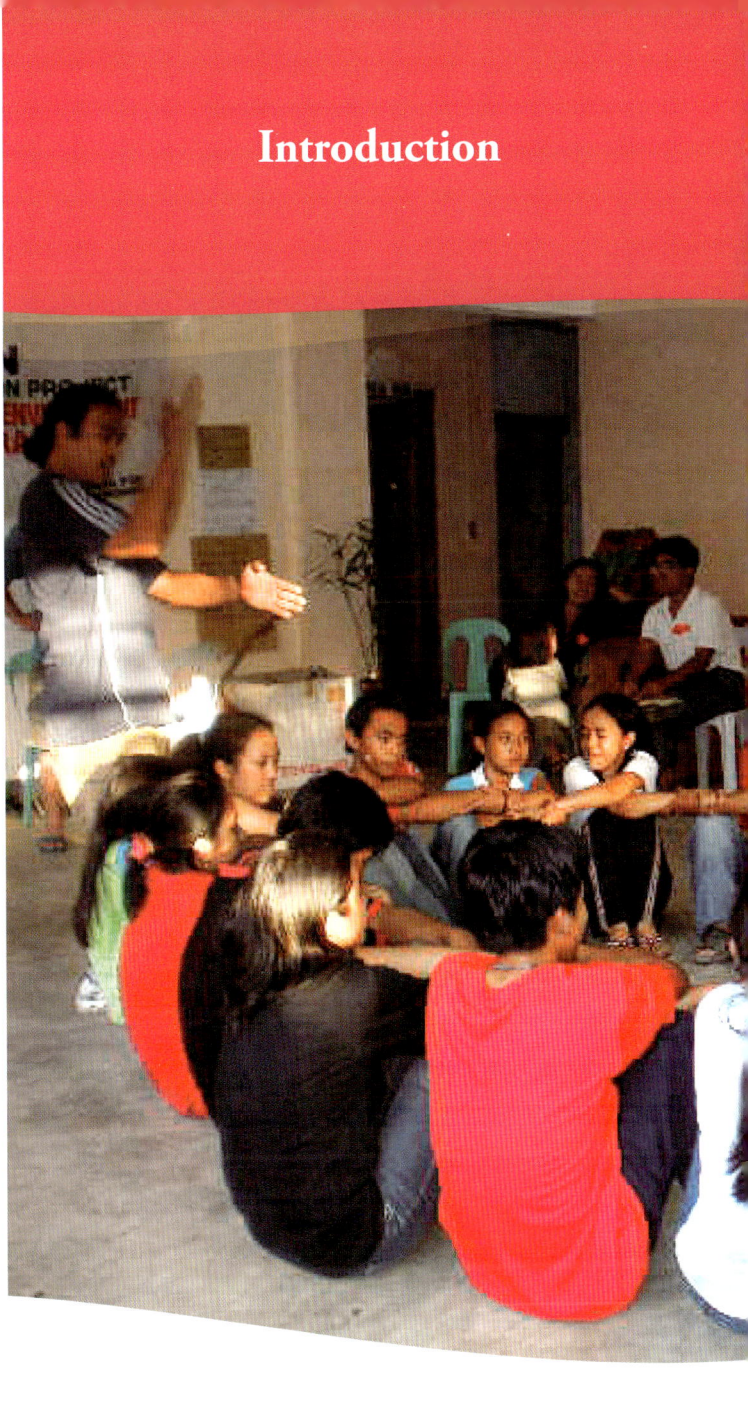

Integrating Poverty and Gender into Health Programmes: *A Sourcebook for Health Professionals*
Module on HIV/AIDS

Introduction

Twenty-five years since the onslaught of the HIV/AIDS epidemic, the number of people infected with the virus continues to rise. Globally, 33.2 million people are living with HIV.[3] In the Region, the epidemic is largely entrenched among marginalized populations, with at least one country, Papua New Guinea, experiencing a generalized epidemic. In some countries, the means of transmission are changing, often exploiting the vulnerability of women and young people to infection.

Experience increasingly shows that the socioeconomic factors contributing to the rapid spread of HIV in the Region include low education, limited access to health care services and increased mobility within and between countries—factors that are largely determined by poverty and gender inequality.[4] For example, evidence from Cambodia and Viet Nam reveal a strong association between poverty and lack of education and an increased risk of infection.[5] Gender inequality enhances the vulnerability of women, particularly young women, to HIV infection, as the rising rates of HIV among women worldwide attest. Evidence similarly shows that poverty and gender inequality can limit the access of poor men and women, boys and girls, to appropriate prevention, diagnosis, treatment and care for HIV/AIDS.

The growing commitment to curbing the HIV/AIDS epidemic requires that health professionals at the community, provincial, national and international level have the knowledge, skills and tools to more effectively respond to the health needs of poor and marginalized people. The need for such knowledge and skills has become more pressing in face of the pledge to ensure universal access to prevention, treatment and care for HIV/AIDS in the Region. However, many health professionals in the Region are not adequately prepared to address these issues.

This module is designed to improve the awareness, knowledge and skills of health professionals on the poverty- and gender-related dimensions of HIV/AIDS. It is divided into six sections:

- **Section 1** provides a brief overview of the HIV/AIDS pandemic and an understanding of HIV and AIDS.
- **Section 2** examines WHAT the links are between poverty, gender and HIV/AIDS.
- **Section 3** discusses WHY it is important for health professionals to address HIV/AIDS, from efficiency, equity and human rights perspectives.
- **Section 4** discusses HOW health professionals can address poverty and gender concerns in HIV/AIDS.
- **Section 5** provides notes for facilitators.
- **Section 6** contains a collection of tools, resources and references to support health professionals in their work in this field.

1. What is HIV/AIDS?

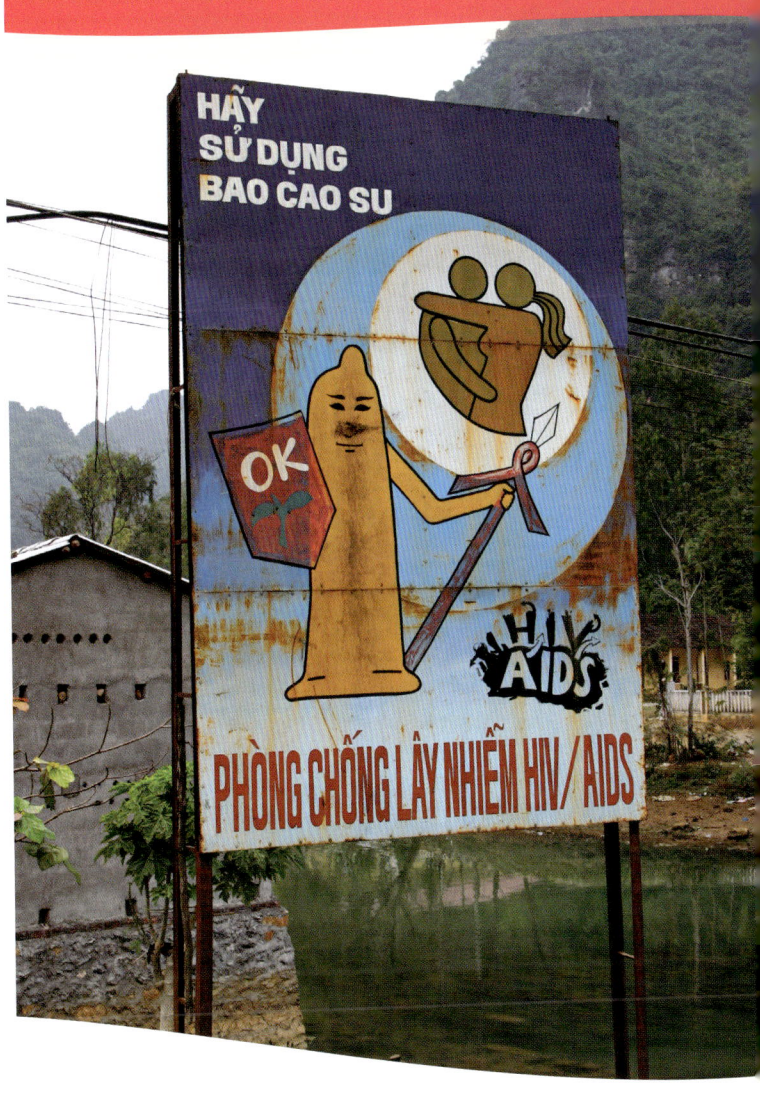

1. What is HIV/AIDS?

The human immunodeficiency virus (HIV) compromises the human immune system and impedes its ability to fight infection. HIV leads to acquired immunodeficiency syndrome (AIDS). Through processes that are still not fully understood, HIV is able to infect key cells (CD4 cells) that coordinate the immune system's fight against infection.[6] This slowly leads to persistent, progressive and profound impairment of the immune system. When the body can no longer fight infection, it is said to have acquired the disease called AIDS. When a person with HIV is diagnosed as having AIDS, this means they have one or more of a defined list of otherwise usually rare illnesses or 'opportunistic infections' and conditions such as cancer.[7] Opportunistic infections are infections that take advantage of the body's weakened immune system.

The virus has two sub-types: HIV-1, the most common type found worldwide, and HIV-2, which is found mostly in West Africa. Both HIV-1 and HIV-2 have the same modes of transmission and are associated with similar opportunistic infections and AIDS.[8] Blood tests or the appearance of certain opportunistic infections indicate that the infection has progressed from HIV to AIDS.[9] Various treatment modalities and combinations of antiretroviral (ARV) therapies can reduce HIV progression and transmission (particularly from mother to child).

HIV transmission can be "horizontal" or "vertical". Horizontal transmission occurs through the following:
1. Sexual intercourse (vaginal, anal and oral) or through contact with infected blood, semen, or cervical and vaginal fluids. This is the most frequent mode of transmission worldwide. HIV can be transmitted from any infected person to his or her sexual partner (man to woman, woman to man, man to man, and woman to woman). The presence of other sexually transmitted infections (STIs) increases the risk of HIV transmission.
2. Blood transfusion or transfusion of blood products (e.g. those obtained from donor blood infected by HIV).
3. Injecting or skin-piercing equipment contaminated with HIV.

Vertical transmission occurs from mother to child during pregnancy, labour and delivery or through breast milk.

HIV cannot be transmitted by coughing or sneezing; handshakes; insect bites; work or school contact; touching, hugging or kissing; using toilets; water or food; using telephones; swimming pools; public baths; or sharing cups, glasses, plates and other eating, drinking or cooking utensils.

WHO clinical staging system for HIV infection and disease

As the use of antiretroviral therapy (ART) increases, surveillance of AIDS alone does not provide adequate information on the magnitude of the HIV epidemic. Information on adults and children with HIV infection is more useful for: estimating the treatment and care burden; planning for effective prevention and care efforts; and assessing care initiatives.[10] In response, WHO recently revised the case definitions for surveillance of HIV and the clinical and immunological classification of HIV-related diseases. The case definition of HIV has been simplified and harmonized with the revised clinical staging and immunological classification that have been updated to facilitate the clinical management of HIV in low-income settings, where the capacity for sophisticated laboratory investigation remains low.

A person with HIV is defined by WHO as "an individual with HIV infection irrespective of clinical stage, confirmed by laboratory criteria according to country definition and requirements".[11] Once HIV infection has been confirmed, the clinical staging system is used. The revised clinical staging system is based on a universal four-stage system. This system outlines the clinical criteria and the definition of symptoms, signs and diseases that determines whether a patient is at clinical stage 1 (asymptomatic), 2 (mild symptoms), 3 (advanced symptoms) or 4 (severe symptoms).[12]

Table 1: WHO clinical staging of HIV/AIDS for adults and adolescents with confirmed HIV infection

Clinical Stage 1

Asymptomatic

Persistent generalized lymphadenopathy

Clinical Stage 2

Unexplained moderate weight loss (<10% of presumed or measured body weight)i

Recurrent respiratory tract infections (sinusitis, tonsillitis, otitis media and pharyngitis)

Herpes zoster

Angular cheilitis

Recurrent oral ulceration

Papular pruritic eruptions

Seborrhoeic dermatitis

Fungal nail infections

Source: World Health Organization 2006c.

Table 1 outlines the clinical conditions categorized under the four stages for adults and adolescents. Confidentiality and security need to guide the collection and reporting of HIV surveillance data. Clinical staging is important as a criterion for starting antiretroviral therapy.

The global burden of HIV/AIDS

Globally, 33.2 million people carry the HIV virus.[13] Each year, about 2.5 million more become infected with HIV. Roughly 2.1 million people died of AIDS in 2007.[14] Unknown a quarter of a century ago, HIV/AIDS is now the leading cause of death and lost years of productive life for adults aged 15–59 years worldwide.[15] Table 2 presents a global summary of the HIV/AIDS epidemic in 2007.

Globally, the incidence rate of HIV appears to have peaked in the late 1990s and has begun to stabilize. Because of the relatively stable incidence rate and the continuing high levels of AIDS-related mortality, the HIV prevalence rate appears to be levelling off since 2001. However, because of population growth and the effect of antiretrovirals (ARVs), the number of people living with HIV is still large.[16]

In many parts of the developing world, most new infections occur in young adults, with young women being especially vulnerable. By 2006, roughly 40% of all adults aged 15 years and over living with HIV/AIDS were young people (15–24 years of age).[17] In sub-Saharan Africa, three women are infected for every two men. Among adults aged 15–44 years of age, the ratio of female to male infection increases to 3:1.[18]

More than 2.5 million children are living with HIV.[19] Every year an estimated 2.2 million pregnant women infected with HIV give birth and, about 700 000 of these newborns contract HIV from their mothers.[20] In addition, AIDS is compounded by the synergy between HIV and tuberculosis (TB). The spread of HIV has contributed to as much as a fourfold increase in the number of persons with TB in parts of Africa. More than 10 million people worldwide are infected with both TB and HIV.[21]

The vast majority of people with HIV/AIDS live in sub-Saharan Africa, ands the crisis continues to grow there. In Asia, an estimated 4.9 million

Table 2: Global summary of the AIDS epidemic

	2001	2007
Number of adults (15+) and children living with HIV	29.0 million (26.9 million–32.4 million)	33.2 million (30.6 million–36.1 million)
Number of adults (15+) and children newly infected with HIV	3.2 million (2.1 million–4.4 million)	2.5 million (1.8 million–4.1 million)
HIV prevalence in adults (15–49)	0.8% (0.7%–0.9%)	0.8% (0.7%–0.9%)
Number of adult (15+) and child deaths due to AIDS	1.7 million (1.6 million–2.3 million)	2.1 million (1.9 million–2.4 million)

Source: Joint United Nations Programme on HIV/AIDS 2007g.

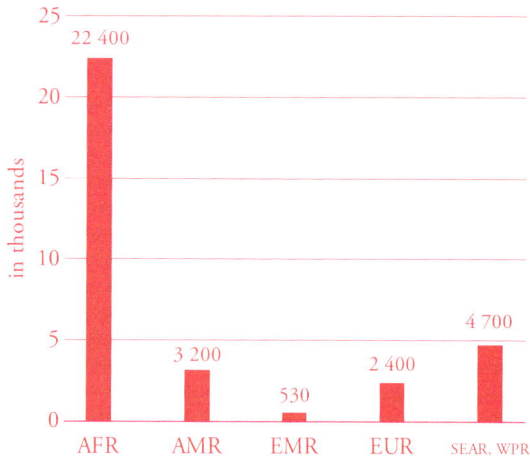

Figure 1: Estimated number of people living with HIV (all ages), by WHO region, 2007

Source: Internal data, from database of UNAIDS/WHO Working Group on Global HIV/AIDS and STI Surveillance, 2007.

people were living with HIV/AIDS in 2007. In the same year, roughly 300 000 adults and children died of AIDS.[22] In the Pacific region, an estimated 81 000 people were living with HIV/AIDS in 2006. The HIV prevalence rate in the Pacific was calculated to be 0.4% in 2006.[23] The proportion of adults living with HIV who are women is 29% in Asia and 47% in the Pacific.[24]

The prevalence of HIV/AIDS in other regions of the world varies considerably, with new infections having declined in Eastern Europe from 230 000 to 150 000 between 2001 and 2007, mainly due to the slower growth of the epidemic in the Russian Federation. In the Caribbean, Latin America, the Middle East and North Africa, North America and Western Europe, the numbers of new HIV infections remained approximately stable between 2001 and 2007.[25] Figure 1 depicts the estimated number of people of all ages living with HIV in 2007, by WHO region.

When estimating the prevalence of HIV within countries, a distinction is made between generalized and concentrated epidemics. In a "generalized epidemic", the adult HIV prevalence exceeds 1% in the general population and HIV transmission mostly occurs through heterosexual sex. In countries with generalized epidemics, the prevalence of HIV is based on surveillance of pregnant women attending antenatal clinics. In the absence of population-based surveys that test for HIV antibodies, this approach provides a good proxy of HIV prevalence in the general population. A "concentrated epidemic" is defined as one in which HIV is concentrated in groups of people whose behaviour exposes them to a high risk of HIV infection. Such epidemics are further categorized into concentrated epidemics, where HIV prevalence is measured as consistently over 5% in at least one defined sub-population and low-level epidemics, where HIV prevalence has not consistently exceeded 5% in any defined sub-population. In these countries, the prevalence

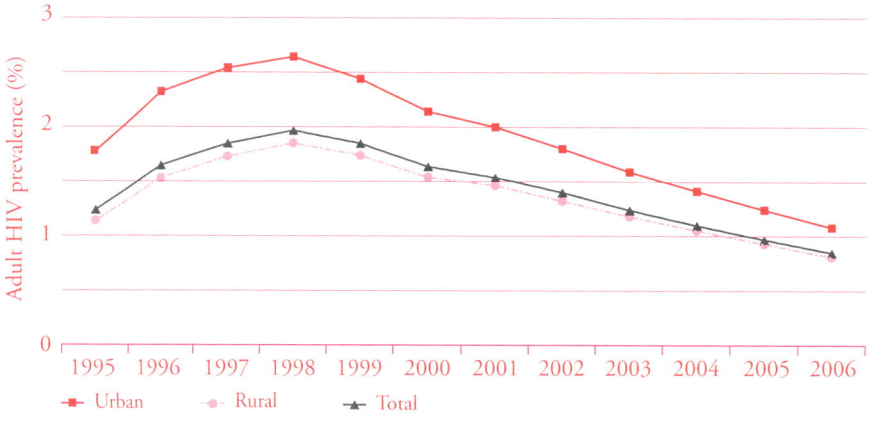

Figure 2: HIV prevalence among the general population in Cambodia, 1995–2006

Source: Joint United Nations Programme on HIV/AIDS and World Health Organization 2007g.

of HIV is based on studies of key populations who are at high risk of HIV exposure, such as injecting drug users (IDUs), sex workers, clients of sex workers and men who have sex with men (MSM).[26]

Many countries in sub-Saharan African are experiencing generalized epidemics. The prevalence of HIV in countries in southern Africa is especially high, with the exception of Angola. South Africa is the country with the largest number of HIV infections in the world, with an estimated 29% of pregnant women infected in 2006.[27]

In the Western Pacific Region, generalized epidemics were previously reported in Cambodia and Papua New Guinea. However, in Cambodia the prevalence of HIV has decreased among the adult population. Figure 2 presents HIV prevalence among the general population in Cambodia from 1995 to 2006. In China, Malaysia and Viet Nam, HIV transmission occurs primarily in vulnerable groups, especially sex workers and their clients, MSM and IDUs.

The nature, pace and severity of HIV epidemics differ across the Western Pacific Region. Overall, Asian countries can be divided into several categories, according to the epidemics they are experiencing. While Cambodia, Myanmar and Thailand were hit early, other countries are only now starting to experience rapidly expanding epidemics. These countries include Indonesia, Nepal, Viet Nam, and several provinces in China. In Myanmar and in parts of India and China, HIV has become entrenched in some sections of the population, despite efforts to halt the spread of the virus. Other countries are still seeing extremely low levels of HIV prevalence, even among people at high risk of exposure to HIV, and therefore have golden opportunities to pre-empt more serious epidemics. These countries include Bangladesh, the Lao People's Democratic Republic, Mongolia, Pakistan, the Philippines and Timor Leste. In the Pacific, the generalized epidemic in Papua New Guinea contrasts with the very low levels of transmission in other Pacific island nations. Table 3 presents HIV estimations for selected countries in the Western Pacific Region, as of 2007.

Table 3: HIV estimations for selected countries in the Western Pacific Region, 2005

Country	HIV estimates in adults (15–49 years)	HIV estimates in women (15–49 years)	AIDS deaths (all ages)	HIV prevalence (%) in adults
Australia	18 000	1 200	<100	0.2
Cambodia	70 000	20 000	6 900	0.8
China	690 000	200 000	39 000	0.1
Fiji	<500	<200	<100	<0.1
Japan	9 600	2 300	<100	<0.1
Lao People's Democratic Republic	5 400	1 300	<100	0.2
Malaysia	79 000	21 000	3 100	0.3
Mongolia	<1 000	<200	<100	0.1
New Zealand	1 400	<500	<100	0.1
Papua New Guinea	53 000	21 000	<1 000	1.5
Philippines	8 200	2 200	<200	<0.1
Republic of Korea	13 000	3 600	<500	<0.1
Singapore	4 100	1 200	<200	0.2
Viet Nam	280 000	76 000	20 000	0.5

Note: IDU, injecting drug user; MSM, men who have sex with men; STI, sexually transmitted infection.
Source: Joint United Nations Programme on HIV/AIDS 2008.

Figure 3: Reported HIV infections by sex, Papua New Guinea, 1987–2006

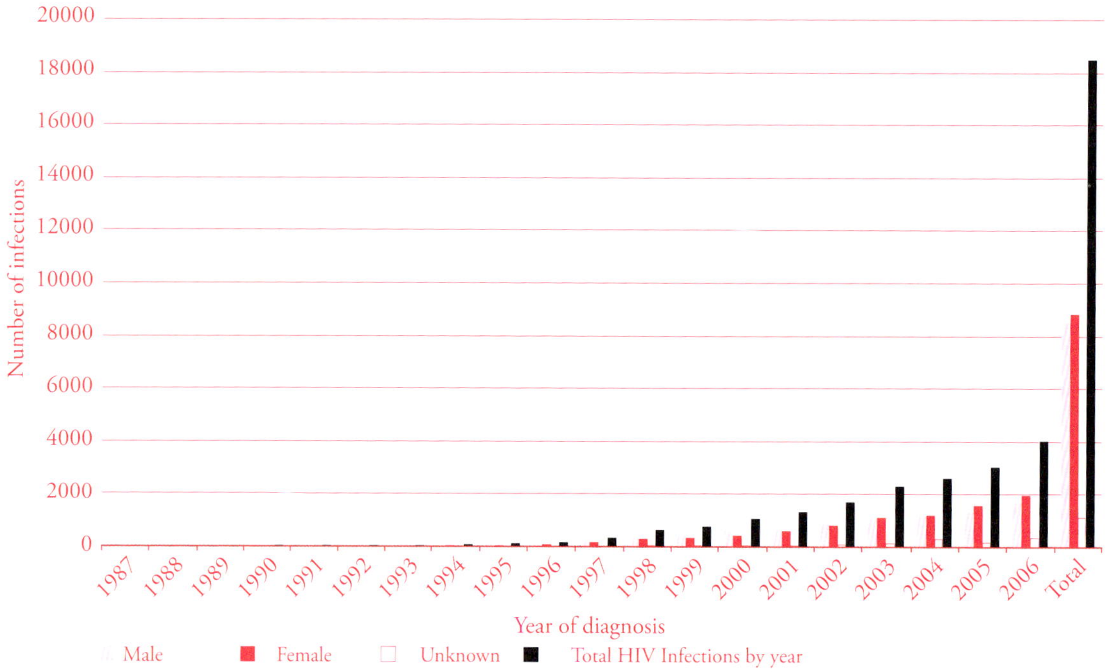

Legend: Male ■ Female □ Unknown ■ Total HIV Infections by year

Source: Government of Papua New Guinea 2007.

Papua New Guinea, which shares an island with one of Indonesia's worst HIV-affected provinces, Papua, has the highest prevalence of HIV infection in the Pacific. An estimated 54 000 Papua New Guineans were living with HIV at the end of 2007.[28] The number of reported HIV infections was much higher among women aged 15–29 years of age than men of the same age, as Figure 3 shows.[29] Young women (15–24 years) appear to be particularly vulnerable, with up to twice as many young women being infected with HIV as men of the same age.[30] Available data suggest the epidemic is centred on commercial and casual sex, most of it heterosexual. High HIV prevalence has been found among sex workers (above 10% in the capital, Port Moresby, for example).

HIV infection levels appear to be very low in other countries in the Pacific, but the data are extremely limited. Table 4 presents the latest estimates for the Pacific.

HIV infection levels in Asian countries in the Western Pacific Region are low compared with countries in other parts of the world, notably those in Africa. But the populations of Asian nations such as China are so large that even low national HIV prevalence rates translate into large numbers of people living with HIV.[31] The estimated number of people living with HIV in Viet Nam more than doubled between 2000 and 2005. As of 2005, HIV had been detected in all 64 of Viet Nam's provinces as well as the major cities. An estimated 80 000 people were living with HIV in Malaysia in 2007, although the prevalence among women seeking antenatal care remains low (0.4% in 2002). The prevalence rate in Cambodia seems to have declined, following its peak in the late 1990s. The national prevalence rates in China and the Philippines remain well under 0.1%, although, as Table 5 shows, China's low prevalence rate coupled with its large population translates into a sizeable number of people living with HIV/AIDS.

In some countries, the means of transmission are changing. In Cambodia, for example, wives of infected men make up nearly half of all new HIV infections; children of infected mothers make up

Table 4: HIV and AIDS statistics and features in the Pacific

	Number of adults and children living with HIV	Number of adults and children newly infected	HIV prevalence in adults	Number of adult and child deaths due to AIDS
2004	72 000 (44 000–150 000)	8000 (39 000–61 000)	0.3%	2900 (1600–4600)
2006	81 000 (50 000–170 000)	7100 (34 000–540 000)	0.4%	4000 (23 000–66 000)

Source: Joint United Nations Programme on HIV/AIDS and World Health Organization 2006a.

one third.[32] In addition, low national prevalence rates in many countries in the Region mask localized epidemics in different areas or vulnerable populations.[33] For example, while HIV has been detected in each of China's provinces, most reported cases are from Guangdong, Guangxi, Henan, Xinjian and Yunnan.[34] Similarly, although the national prevalence rate remains below 0.1%, just under half of people living with HIV are estimated to have been infected while injecting drugs. HIV prevalence has been found to exceed 50% among IDUs in some areas of Xinjiang, Yunnan and Sichuan provinces.[35] The results of sentinel surveillance show that the prevalence of HIV among IDUs was 6.48% in 2004.[36] An estimated 89.5% of IDUs dwell in just seven provinces (Guangdong, Guangxi, Guizhou, Hunan, Sichuan, Xinjiang and Yunnan).[37] The prevalence of HIV among pregnant women is estimated to range from 0.3% to 1.6% in Yunnan province. In Henan and Xinjiang provinces, HIV prevalence rates above 1% have been observed among pregnant women and women receiving premarital and clinical HIV testing. The epidemic has begun to spread from these vulnerable groups to the general population in some areas in China and Cambodia.[38] Among other vulnerable groups, infection rates in men who have sex with men have begun to rise in Cambodia, China, Mongolia and Viet Nam.[39]

Table 5: Estimated number of people with HIV/AIDS in China

Epidemiological data	2007
Number of adults (15+) living with HIV	690 000 (450 000–1 000 000)
AIDS-related deaths	39 000 (23 000–62 000)
Number of women living with HIV	200 000 (120 000–310 000)

Source: Joint United Nations Programme on HIV/AIDS 2008.

2. What are the links between poverty, gender and HIV/AIDS?

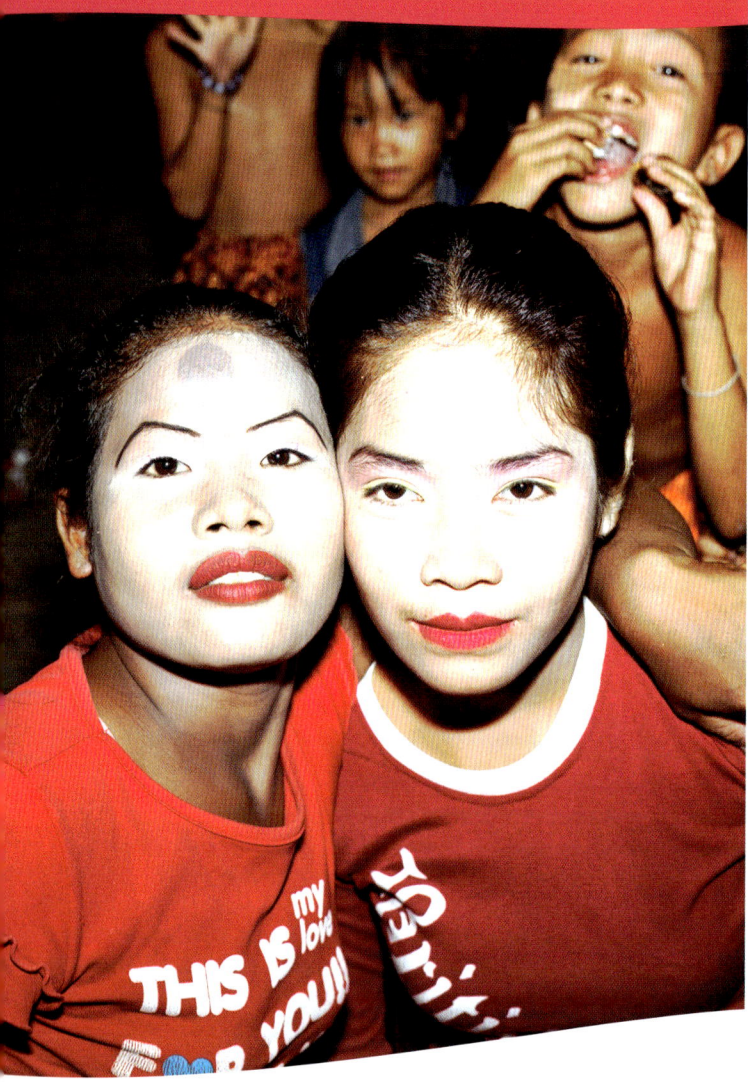

Integrating Poverty and Gender into Health Programmes: *A Sourcebook for Health Professionals*
Module on HIV/AIDS

2. What are the links between poverty, gender and HIV/AIDS?

Over the last decades, we have learned that the HIV epidemic is fuelled by poverty, lack of education and gender inequality.

- Joint United Nations Programme on HIV/AIDS 2002a

The relationship between HIV/AIDS, poverty and gender is complex. Poor people usually have lower access to health services including those for effective treatment of sexually transmitted infections (STIs), HIV/AIDS prevention and treatment, or prevention of mother-to-child transmission (PMTCT).[40] In addition, poor people may be less likely to seek health care for opportunistic infections, and may often access health services only in the later stages of the disease, due to various barriers to access to services. As a result, for a poor person with HIV/AIDS, the time between the first presentation at a health care centre and death is often very short.[41]

This section discusses these issues. To achieve a better understanding of the relationship between HIV/AIDS, poverty and gender, two lines of enquiry are considered: (1) how poverty- or gender-related factors increase the probability of HIV infection and progression from HIV to AIDS, as well as morbidity and mortality from opportunistic infections; and (2) how AIDS may cause or increase poverty or exacerbate gender inequalities.[42]

This section begins by considering the relationship between poverty and HIV/AIDS. Box 1 outlines how poverty is conceptualized in this module.[43]

The links between poverty and HIV/AIDS

The relationship between poverty and HIV/AIDS is multifaceted and likely works along a number of interrelated and overlapping pathways. While many of these pathways remain opaque, it is increasingly clear that the links between poverty and HIV/AIDS can run in both directions. That is, poverty in its multiple dimensions can influence the likelihood of HIV infection, progression to full blown AIDS, and AIDS-related mortality. This occurs through poor nutrition, limited education and restricted access to appropriate diagnosis, treatment and care, among other factors. Conversely, people with HIV/AIDS are likely to experience greater poverty as a result of reduced labour productivity when ill and the costs of treatment and care, which may drain the resources of already poor households. The loss of a productive family member to AIDS may reduce household income over the short to medium term with longer-term implications for children in the household,

---

Box 1: Defining poverty

In this module, poverty is defined as encompassing not only low income or consumption but also other forms of deprivation, including limited economic opportunities; diminished education and health outcomes; reduced access to services, resources and skills; and voicelessness and powerlessness to influence decisions that affect one's life. This definition moves beyond a narrow conceptualization of poverty as comprising low income and consumption, which tends to inadequately capture the experience of poverty in the Region. For example, among communities in the Pacific, levels of income or consumption poverty are often low or nonexistent. However, households in the Pacific can be vulnerable to natural disasters; be isolated or remote; lack economic choices (or opportunities to earn a cash income); have limited access to educational, health and financial services; and suffer from social exclusion.[44]

Poverty often overlaps with and reinforces other types of social exclusions such as those based on age, ethnicity, geographical location and gender. Because of this, communities, households and even members within the same household tend to have different experiences of poverty. The poverty experienced in rural communities often differs in important ways from that of urban poor communities, such as slum dwellers. Women within poor households tend to be particularly disadvantaged, as women lag behind men in almost every social and economic indicator of well-being.[45]

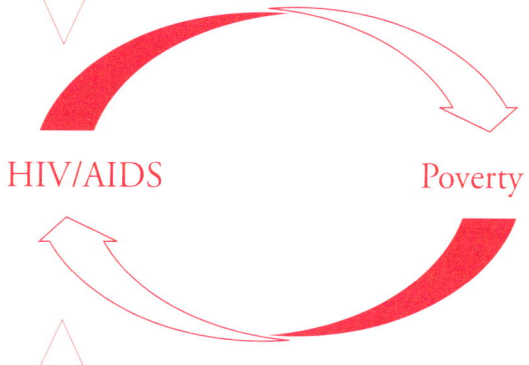

Figure 4: The relationship between poverty and HIV/AIDS

- Structural vulnerability → high-risk situations
- Lack of access to preventive interventions
- Lack of access to affordable care
- Lower educational status → reduced access to information on AIDS

HIV/AIDS ⇄ Poverty

- Lost productivity
- Catastrophic costs of health care
- Increased dependency ratio
- Orphans with worse nutrition, lower school enrolment
- Decreased capacity to manage households headed by orphans, elderly
- Reduced national income
- Fewer national resources for HIV/AIDS control

Source: Adeyi et al. 2001.

through the intergenerational transmission of poverty. Figure 4 depicts the relationship between poverty and HIV/AIDS.

Figure 4 outlines a number of the pathways through which the links between poverty and HIV/AIDS likely operate. As yet, evidence is insufficient to make the assertion that poverty causes AIDS. However, as the evidence base mounts, the mechanisms through which poverty can increase vulnerability to HIV infection and the progression from HIV to AIDS and AIDS-related mortality are slowly being illuminated. At present, some pathways through which poverty may lead to HIV/AIDS have been demonstrated; others remain unclear and poorly understood.[46]

At this time, it is probably too simplistic to portray HIV/AIDS as a disease of the poor. For example, in many countries, the urban elite are the ones purchasing sex, while travelling business people and officers in the armed forced are having casual sex. These men (and women) are vulnerable to HIV transmission, yet they are not poor.[47] However, the relationship between poverty and HIV/AIDS is likely dynamic, changing as the HIV/AIDS epidemic in the Region progresses. Improved evidence will likely shed more light on this relationship and the pathways of concern at the household, community and national levels.

Analysis of available data suggests that the relationship between poverty and HIV/AIDS may operate at the global, regional, national and local levels, although this relationship has been more clearly analysed at some levels than at others.[48] At the local or individual level, the multiple dimensions of poverty, such as lower educational level, fewer livelihood choices, and reduced capacity to negotiate safe sex, probably increase the risk of becoming HIV-infected. For example, as the sections below discuss, evidence suggests that improved education and knowledge of HIV/AIDS can reduce the probability of HIV infection. Once infected, economic and social costs may delay seeking diagnosis, treatment and care for HIV/AIDS and may increase the likelihood of progression from HIV infection to AIDS, as well as of death from opportunistic infections.

In most countries in the Region, the epidemic is largely concentrated within marginalized groups which, while not always income- or consumption-poor, are likely to experience discrimination that can heighten their vulnerability to HIV/AIDS. Globally, the distribution of HIV/AIDS has been positively associated with absolute poverty.[49]

The sections below outline the evidence on the ways in which poverty can increase the likelihood of HIV infection and progression to AIDS and AIDS-related mortality. The section begins with an overview of the association between poverty and HIV at the global, national and local levels.

The effect of poverty on HIV infection

Developing countries are home to an estimated 85% of the global population and more than 95% of HIV-infected people.[50] Sub-Saharan Africa, which bears the brunt of the global HIV/AIDS epidemic, has the lowest gross national product (GNP) of any region in the world.[51] Analysis of cross-country evidence has revealed a significant positive association between high HIV prevalence and low socioeconomic performance. This relationship was found to hold true regardless of the measure of socioeconomic performance used, be it per capita income, income inequality, absolute poverty or the UNDP Human Poverty Index.[52]

While the association between poverty and HIV appears to have been demonstrated at the global level, the picture at the regional and national levels remains less clear. A study of poverty and HIV concluded that no clear relationship exists between poverty and national rates of HIV in any continent, including Asia. The notable exception was Africa, which reported a negative correlation between socioeconomic status and HIV.[53] A study in 1999 found that the prevalence of HIV was higher among people who were better educated and wealthier than among those who were poor and less educated.[54] The results of more recent research suggest that this negative association between HIV and poverty in Africa may have lessened. Analysis of population survey data carried out in 2006 concluded that no correlation exists between education level and HIV status.[55]

Initially, HIV may disproportionately affect people who were wealthy and well educated. However, the growing consensus is that, as the epidemic progresses, the incidence of HIV becomes increasingly concentrated in poor and marginalized populations.[56] In addition to the evidence cited from the African region, this assertion is supported by evidence from Brazil. In the early 1980s, an estimated 75% of people who were newly diagnosed with HIV in Brazil had a secondary education or higher. By the early 1990s, this proportion fell to roughly one third.[57] This also seems to be the case in developed countries, where poor and marginalized communities bear a disproportionate burden of HIV.[58] Over time, it is expected that wealthier and better educated populations will be able to protect themselves better from HIV infection and will have greater access to technological innovations, such as ART, which will enable them to lead productive and healthy lives. In contrast, poor populations, which tend to have less access to information and appropriate treatment and care for HIV/AIDS, will be unable or unwilling to protect themselves from HIV infection because of hardship and destitution.

Notwithstanding the lack of a statistically significant (positive or negative) association between national HIV prevalence rates and poverty in Asia, a brief review of available data suggests that the burden of HIV/AIDS in the Western Pacific Region is largely concentrated among developing countries. Papua New Guinea and, previously Cambodia, the two countries with generalized epidemics in the Region, are classified as low-income economies.[59] The prevalence of HIV is expanding rapidly in other low- and lower-middle-income economies in the Region, such as Viet Nam and China. To date, the prevalence rate in upper-middle-income economies, such

---

Box 2: Populations vulnerable to HIV/AIDS

People living in poverty
People with low levels of education
People living in remote regions
Women
Ethnic minorities
Youths and infants
Sex workers
Infecting drug users
People engaged in skin piercing, e.g. tattoos
Blood donors and recipients of blood or organ transplants
Prisoners or people in other types of closed settings
Refugees
Migrant workers
Military and police personnel
Internally displaced populations (due to war, famine, earthquake, other natural disasters, civil unrest, etc.)

Figure 5: Poverty increases the likelihood of HIV infection and AIDS

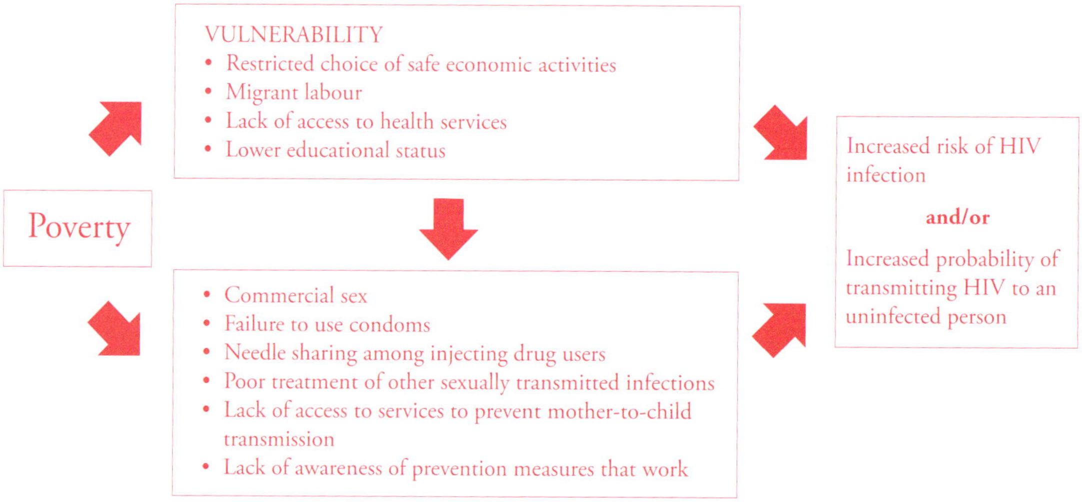

Poverty →

VULNERABILITY
- Restricted choice of safe economic activities
- Migrant labour
- Lack of access to health services
- Lower educational status

- Commercial sex
- Failure to use condoms
- Needle sharing among injecting drug users
- Poor treatment of other sexually transmitted infections
- Lack of access to services to prevent mother-to-child transmission
- Lack of awareness of prevention measures that work

→ Increased risk of HIV infection

and/or

Increased probability of transmitting HIV to an uninfected person

Source: Adeyi *et al.* 2001.

as Malaysia and the Philippines, has remained relatively low.

A number of countries in the Region are experiencing localized epidemics in certain geographical areas, vulnerable populations and specific age groups. For example, seven of the 10 provinces in China with a high prevalence rate of HIV are located in the economically underdeveloped central and western regions.[60] Box 2 lists populations that have been identified as being particularly vulnerable to HIV/AIDS, although the vulnerability differs across the different groups.

Often, discussion of HIV infection in these populations focuses on the role of high-risk behaviours in the transmission of the virus. Focusing on individual behaviour obscures the fact that people act within a context that is shaped by economic, political and cultural elements within a society, which can increase the vulnerability of some people to HIV infection.[61] For example, poverty may reduce an individual's ability or willingness to take actions considered necessary to avoid infection. Poverty may also increase the likelihood that people will engage in high-risk occupations, such as sex work. Poverty is further associated with lower educational attainment, which in turn is linked with lower awareness of effective measures to prevent HIV infection.[62] Figure 5 presents various ways in which poverty can be understood to lead to increased risk of HIV infection.

A growing body of evidence confirms the links between poverty and HIV infection at the household (micro) level. The sections below consider various pathways through which poverty can increase the vulnerability of individuals to HIV/AIDS infection.

Low household income

Studies from a number of countries in Asia have reported an association between low household income and increased likelihood of HIV infection. For example, research carried out in Thailand found that people from the poorest households in the study population were the most likely to be infected with HIV.[63] Similarly, in India, low household socioeconomic status significantly contributed to the likelihood of people being infected with HIV.[64] Low household income was also associated with increased risk of infection in Sri Lanka.[65] Similarly, household income has been

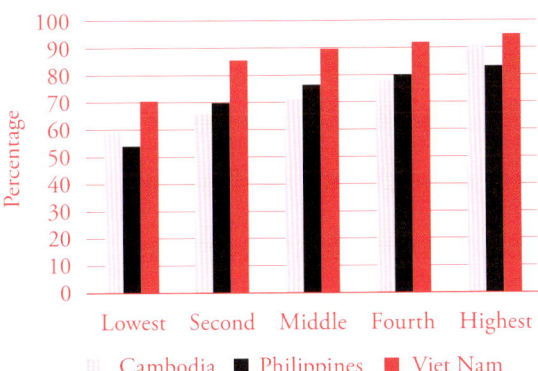

Figure 6: Proportion of women aged 15–49 years who know at least one way to avoid sexual transmission of HIV by income quintile, in Cambodia (2000), the Philippines (2003) and Viet Nam (2002)

Source: Gwatkin D. *et al.* 2007a, b and c.

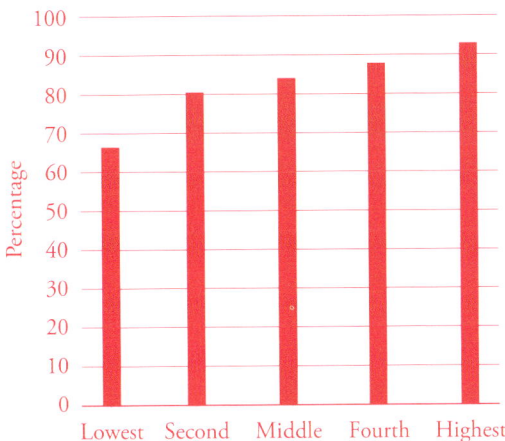

Figure 7: Proportion of men aged 15–54 years who know at least one way to avoid sexual transmission of HIV, by income quintile, in the Philippines

Source: Gwatkin *et al.* 2007b.

positively correlated with reduced risk factors for HIV, such as increased awareness of modern contraceptives and the benefit of condoms, in Cambodia and Viet Nam.[66] Evidence suggests that women's awareness of HIV prevention methods improves as household income rises in Cambodia, the Philippines and Viet Nam (Figure 6); men's awareness also improves in the Philippines (Figure 7).

While these data suggest that the protective effect of higher household income may operate through improved education and knowledge of HIV, further analysis of the Cambodian and Vietnamese data concluded that household income and education also have independent effects on reduced risk factors for HIV. This may be because people living in poor households are less able to afford preventive measures, such as condoms. Similarly, low household income may be associated with many of the other factors outlined below.

Geographical location

In many countries in the Region, poverty is largely concentrated in rural communities. The percentage of the poor residing in rural areas is 90% in Cambodia, 94% in the Philippines and 74% in Viet Nam.[67] In the Lao People's Democratic Republic, the poverty rate in urban areas was estimated at 27%, compared with 41% in rural areas.[68]

The burden of HIV in countries in the Region may be unevenly distributed between urban and rural areas. In some countries, IDUs, sex workers and MSM, among other populations vulnerable to HIV, tend to reside in urban rather than rural areas. However, according to the World Bank, because the populations of many developing countries remain largely rural, the number of people living with HIV may actually be higher in rural areas.[69] China's experience of HIV may be unique, in that the epidemic spread from rural to urban areas. An estimated 70% of people infected with HIV in China live in rural communities.[70] Notably, in China, transmission in the early stages of the epidemic occurred mostly through faulty plasma collection procedures. High rates of STI have been reported in rural and remote communities in some Pacific island countries. In Papua New Guinea, for example, a study estimated that 59% of women in a small village in Asaro Valley in the Eastern Highlands Province had an STI in 1998.[71] Interestingly, a study found HIV prevalence to be twice as high among sex workers in a rural province in Cambodia as among sex workers in Phnom Penh. The study suggested that the comparatively older age of sex workers in rural areas may have resulted in higher rates of HIV.[72]

In countries where the incidence of HIV has clustered in urban areas, it is possible that rural communities are uniquely vulnerable to HIV transmission. This vulnerability is likely a result of the generally poor coverage of health care facilities in rural areas and inadequate prevention and surveillance efforts. In addition, migration patterns and the tendency for HIV-positive people in urban areas to return to their rural communities when they fall ill will tend to influence the shape of the HIV epidemic in rural communities.

Knowledge and awareness of HIV/AIDS has also been found to be lower among rural communities. A study of knowledge of HIV/AIDS among college students attending university in Beijing and Nanjing, China, concluded that students from urban areas had significantly higher levels of knowledge of HIV than those from rural areas.[73] The proportion of women aged 15–49 years who knew at least one way to avoid the sexual transmission of HIV was calculated to be 86% in urban areas as compared with 71% in rural areas of Cambodia. Similarly, women of the same age group in urban areas were more likely to know that HIV/AIDS can be transmitted from mother to child than were women from rural areas (85.3% vs. 69.6%).[74] A similar pattern was observed in the Philippines and Viet Nam.[75] In the Philippines, the proportion of men aged 15–54 years who used a condom the last time they had sex with a non-regular partner was found to be 31.0% in urban areas and 28.6% in rural areas in 2003.[76]

Lower educational status

Poor people often have lower levels of education and less access to educational messages about HIV than those who are better-off. There is growing evidence that lower educational status and illiteracy lead to a lack of awareness about HIV/AIDS and its modes of transmission.[77] In Bangladesh, Nepal and Viet Nam, knowledge that condoms can prevent the transmission of HIV was found to be positively correlated with educational attainment. Women with no education were significantly less likely than those with primary school education to know about the preventive effect of condoms, while women with even higher levels of education had the greatest awareness.[78]

Lower awareness of HIV/AIDS has, in turn, been linked with an increased likelihood of risky behaviour. A study in Thailand observed that men with a good understanding of appropriate prevention strategies and the mechanisms of infection were less likely to frequent sex workers than men who had a weak understanding of these issues. A poorer understanding of HIV prevention and transmission was more common among men of lower socioeconomic status.[79] Table 6 presents the findings of a study on the links between poverty, low education and risk-taking behaviour in Viet Nam.

The findings suggest the potentially powerful protective effect of education. For example, high school or higher education attainment

Table 6: Poverty, low education and risk-taking behaviour in Viet Nam

	Wealthiest income quintile (Number of times more likely to be aware of prevention measures compared to those in lower income brackets)	Highest education (Number of times more likely to be aware of prevention measures compared to those with lower education levels)
Condom use	2.684	6.455
Having only one sex partner	1.959	4.144
Avoiding sex with sex workers	2.233	0.967
Knowledge of source of condoms	2.175	34.132
Knowledge about condoms	2.504	26.720

Source: Bloom *et al*. 2001:14 In: Australian Agency for International Development and United Nations Development Programme 2005.

was associated with a lower prevalence of HIV among injecting drug users in Long An Province, Viet Nam, in 2002.[80] However, even when information about HIV/AIDS reaches poor individuals, they may not understand the messages or may not perceive the risk to be important within their day-to-day struggle for survival and thus, may fail to take preventive measures.[81]

Restricted choice of safe economic activities

The income-earning opportunities available to poor people are often restricted by their low levels of education and skills. Faced with limited economic opportunities, the short-term survival needs of poor men and women and their families may lead to the adoption of a range of coping strategies with negative implications for their health and well-being in the medium or longer term.[82] This includes income-earning activities that may increase the risk of poor men and women to HIV infection. For example, while women engage in commercial sex for a variety of reasons, many sex workers are likely to be poor. A study carried out in Siem Reap, Cambodia, found that 51.4% of female sex workers had never attended school.[83]

While a range of income-earning opportunities may increase the vulnerability of poor men and women to HIV infection, much attention has been devoted to the role of migration in the transmission of HIV in the Region. Men and women migrate for a range of reasons. Some migrate in search of improved economic opportunities, while others are tricked or forced into migrating. The vulnerability of economic migrants to HIV infection may differ from those who are forced to migrate or are trafficked. On the other hand, in some cases, the vulnerability of poor economic migrants who have few opportunities, or those who are undocumented in their area or country of residence, may not differ substantially from those who are trafficked. Work-related migration might take place within the country (internal) to rural or urban areas or outside the country of origin.

The positive relationship between migrant labour flows and the spread of HIV is quite strong. Evidence shows that migrants have higher rates of HIV than non-mobile populations, regardless of the HIV prevalence rates at the source or destination sites.[84] A number of factors that contribute to the spread of HIV among labour migrants have been identified. Of particular importance are: length of time away from the social norms of the migrant's home environment; accommodation with members of the same sex; constrained access to reproductive health services; loneliness- and boredom-induced alcohol and drug abuse; and "a dysfunctional symbiosis between migrant labour and sex work".[85] For example, a study in Sichuan province, China, reported that migrant workers constituted the majority of men purchasing sex from female sex workers. On average, migrant workers were found to have bought sex 11 times during the previous six months and the majority (64%) had not used a condom the last time they paid for sex.[86] A study was carried out in 1998 among first-time departing migrant workers in the Philippines to identify the factors that increased their vulnerability to HIV/AIDS. The findings suggest that vulnerability to HIV/AIDS among Filipino migrant workers was linked to low knowledge of HIV/AIDS, limited condom use, poor health-seeking behaviour and a sense of invincibility towards HIV/AIDS. In addition, the study noted that the general neglect of issues such as loneliness, cultural adaptation and possibly difficult working conditions among the study population may have also contributed to their vulnerability.[87]

The following examples, including those from the Region, point to the links between mobility and HIV/AIDS:[88]

- **Migrant workers**: Of the Filipinos reported to be living with HIV, 33% were migrant workers who have returned home. Roughly 75% of these workers were men.[89] About 41% of HIV-positive Bangladeshis were migrant workers. In Shanghai, China, an estimated 60% of people infected with HIV are migrants.[90]

- **Mobile professions**: Research carried out among truck drivers at five South African truck stops revealed an overall HIV/AIDS prevalence rate of 56%, well above the national adult prevalence rate. Fishermen account for 7.8% of people with HIV/AIDS with known occupation in Malaysia and are thus considered to be vulnerable to HIV/AIDS.[91] A cross-sectional STI prevalence survey conducted among seafarers in Kiribati found a high prevalence of chlamydial infection and low rates of condom use with sexual partners in Kiribati and abroad.[92]

- **Migrant and trafficked sex workers**: The sex industry is closely linked with the transmission of HIV in Cambodia. Many female sex workers in Cambodia have been lured from rural areas to large towns and cities with the promise of honest and well-paid jobs. While most female sex workers are Khmer, women from other countries, especially Viet Nam, have migrated or been trafficked to Cambodia.[93] Women and girls who are trafficked tend to be extremely poor.[94]

- **Partners of migrant workers**: In the Philippines, seafarers have been identified as a group that may potentially transmit HIV infections from vulnerable populations, such as sex workers living in port cities in other countries, to the general population.[95]

Many migrant workers return home after periods away. Since much migration originates in rural areas, returning migrants may contribute to the spread of HIV in rural populations.[96] Moreover, when migrant workers in urban areas become ill, they frequently return to their rural villages to be cared for by their families. This return migration places additional pressure on scarce household resources.

Generalized conclusions about diverse migrant populations and their vulnerability to HIV/AIDS need to be made with care. The general view in China, for example, is that migrant workers figure prominently in the growing HIV/AIDS epidemic. While much of the migrant population in China appears to be vulnerable to HIV/AIDS because they are single, separated from their spouse or engaging in high-risk behaviour, this is not always the case. Many men migrant workers move with their women partners. Also, up to one half of migrant workers are women, who tend to engage in risky behaviour less than their male counterparts.[97] The variability in living and working conditions of migrant workers from the Philippines has been associated with their varying vulnerability to HIV infection.[98] The most vulnerable group of migrant workers are those working in the entertainment and sex industry. Live-in domestic workers can also be more vulnerable to HIV, as they tend to be more isolated and dependent upon their employers for access to information and health care than migrant workers who live independently. A study from the Republic of Korea reported varying levels of education, knowledge of HIV/AIDS and risky behaviours among migrant workers from different countries in the Region.[99]

Racial or ethnic minorities

People from ethnic minority groups have been identified as being particularly vulnerable to HIV.[100] Estimates from 2002 suggest that while people from ethnic minority groups in China constitute only about 8% of the population, they account for 36% of HIV infections.[101] Prior to 1995, roughly 77% of HIV infections in the province of Yunnan, China, occurred among the minority Jingpo and Dai peoples.[102] The overrepresentation of ethnic minorities among those with HIV has slowly shifted in Yunnan. In 2004, people from the Jingpao and Dai groups accounted for 9% and 7% of new HIV infection, respectively.[103] These ethnic groups constitute an estimated 0.3% and 2.5% of the general population in Yunnan, respectively.

A study in the United States of America found that African American and Latina women, who make up only 25% of the female population, represent 77% of AIDS cases among women.[104] Several factors accounted for the disproportionate HIV morbidity, including: racial/ethnic group affiliation; socioeconomic status; overall health; sexual risk taking; and higher rates of STI.[105] A recent study reported that a woman's HIV risk was not a function of her race/ethnicity, but more likely attributable to differences in socioeconomic status, exposure to violence, and exposure to risky sexual behaviours.[106] Lack of employment and education opportunities, and the material and psychological benefits that accrue as a result of these, may be more important factors than ethnicity in increasing the risk of HIV transmission.

Evidence shows that levels of education and knowledge of HIV/AIDS vary across ethnic groups in the Region. A study in Xieng Khuang and Oudomxay provinces of the Lao People's Democratic Republic found that HIV/AIDS awareness varied from 53.00% among the Tai-Kadai people to 34.86% among the Khmou people and 9.77% among those from the Hmong ethnic group.[107] A study of behaviour that increases the risk of HIV infection was carried out in Quang Ninh province, Viet Nam. The study covered participants aged 15 to 45 years of age in a rural district (Yen Hung), a mountainous district inhabited largely by ethnic minority groups (Binh Lieu) and an urban district (Ha Long). The study found that the level of education of participants was much lower in Binh Lieu than in the other two districts. An estimated 67% of respondents in Binh Lieu had less than six years of education, as compared with 27% and 2% in Yen Huang and Ha Long, respectively. Similarly, more than 90% of respondents in Yen Huang and Ha Long had heard of HIV as compared with 61% in Binh Lieu.

In some cases, this difference extends to people from religious minorities, too. For example, the proportion of women and men who had heard of HIV and AIDS in the Autonomous Region of Muslim Mindanao (ARMM) in the Philippines, was reported to be 76% and 51.4%, respectively, as compared with 95% and 96% in the general population. An even lower proportion of women and men in ARMM knew about HIV prevention methods.[108]

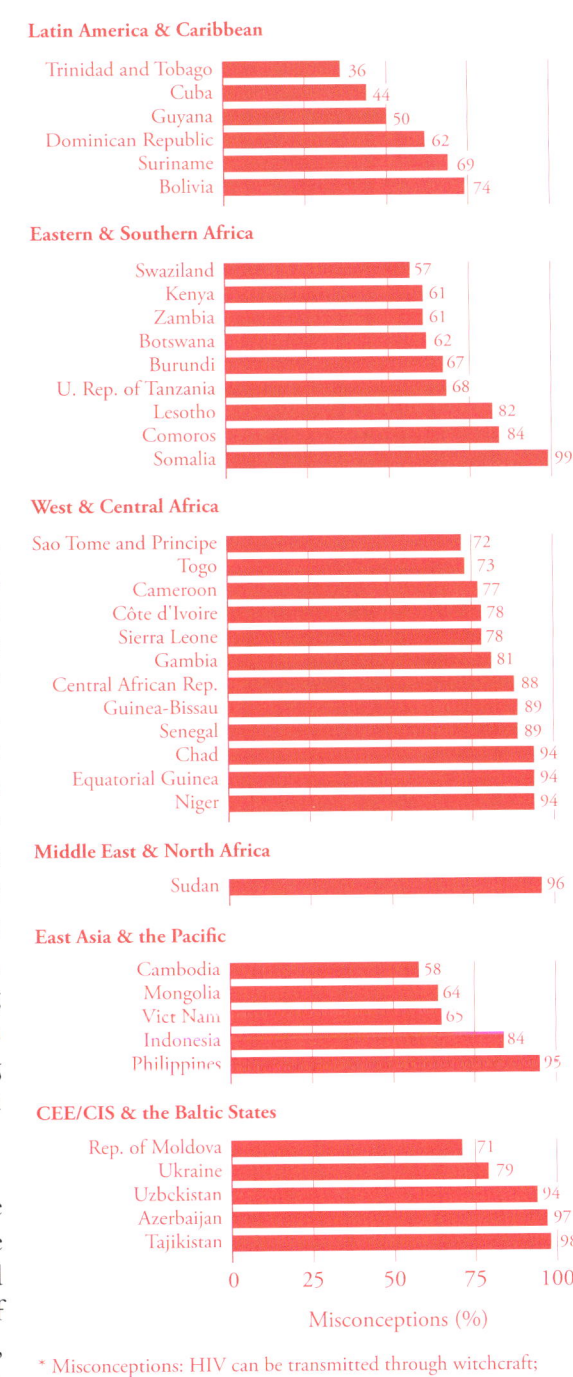

Figure 8: Proportion of girls aged 15–19 years who have at least one major misconception* about HIV/AIDS or had never heard of AIDS, 1999–2001

* Misconceptions: HIV can be transmitted through witchcraft; HIV can be transmitted through mosquito bites; a healthy-looking person cannot have the AIDS virus.
Source: UNICEF/Multiple Indicator Cluster Survey, Measure DHS, 1999–2001. In: United Nations Children's Fund, Joint United Nations Programme on HIV/AIDS and World Health Organization 2002.

What are the links between poverty, gender and HIV/AIDS?

Vulnerability of young people and children

Young people and children have been identified as being particularly vulnerable to HIV. Evidence shows that knowledge about STI and HIV prevention among young people is generally low, increasing their vulnerability to contracting and transmitting STIs and HIV/AIDS. Ignorance and misconceptions concerning HIV/AIDS are common among young people (Figure 8).[109] A nationwide survey of young people aged 15–24 years in the Philippines showed that, although 95% of respondents had heard of HIV/AIDS, over 25% believed that AIDS is curable and 73.4% believed they were not vulnerable to contracting HIV in the future. In addition, roughly 66% of respondents were aware of other STIs.[110] A study of unmarried young people aged 15–24 years in five mountainous provinces of Viet Nam reported that only 24.2% of male and 32.2% of female respondents were able to answer two questions on prevention of the sexual transmission of HIV and dispel major misconceptions about HIV transmission.[111] An estimated 37% of girls aged 15–24 years in Cambodia had comprehensive knowledge of HIV.[112]

Poverty and family disruption can put children and young people at greater risk for HIV/AIDS. Orphaned children may face particular vulnerability. Young people living in poverty, or those facing the threat of poverty, may be especially vulnerable to sexual exploitation through the need to trade or sell sex in order to survive. Estimates suggest that as many as 100 million young people under the age of 18 live or work on the streets of urban areas throughout the world. Many are at heightened risk of acquiring an STI including HIV. Street children in Jakarta, Indonesia, reported that being forced to have sex was one of the greatest problems they faced.[113] Among street children in Viet Nam, roughly 15% are estimated to be HIV positive.[114]

HIV/AIDS and older people

Older people who are sexually active are also at risk for HIV transmission. Yet there is a general lack of understanding about sexuality in older age and that a substantial number of older people remain sexually active. In Thailand, nearly 5% of HIV infections were found to occur among those aged 60 and above in 2002, and the actual prevalence is believed to be higher.[115]

Progression from HIV to AIDS

A poor person who becomes infected with HIV will likely progress from HIV seropositivity to full blown AIDS more rapidly than someone who is better-off. This may occur for a variety of reasons. Poor individuals may be malnourished, thereby increasing vulnerability to infection. Also, a poor person may have limited or delayed access to diagnosis, treatment and care for HIV/AIDS because of financial and non-financial barriers that restrict access to health services. Separately and together, these barriers can delay or prevent the poor from accessing appropriate health services.

The following section considers the geographical, economic and sociocultural barriers to health care. It then discusses inequalities in the quality of treatment and care for HIV/AIDS. Even when the poor are able to access treatment and care, the quality of care is often lower in health facilities serving poor communities than in those in better-off areas. However, experience with treatment for HIV/AIDS in countries in the Region is relatively recent and the evidence base on the access of poor people to ART remains thin. The little available evidence on adherence to ART is discussed in the final section.

Geographical access

Poor individuals dwelling in rural or remote communities often have lower access to adequate health services than their urban counterparts. The coverage of health services in rural and remote areas across the Region remains low and services are often inadequate, including those for reproductive health. An estimated 80% of the population of the Lao People's Democratic Republic, for example, resides in rural areas, mostly in remote villages that are hard to access.

The coverage of health services in Viet Nam is similarly lower in rural than in urban areas. In urban areas in Viet Nam, an estimated 81.0% of pregnant women have three or more visits to a medically trained professional as compared with 53.5% of women in rural areas.[116] A study carried out in a rural community in Papua New Guinea found that although 43.0% of women in the study population reported symptoms related to reproductive track infections, only 9.3% had sought treatment for these symptoms in the previous three months.[117] In Cambodia, HIV/AIDS prevention efforts were found to largely focus on urban populations, thereby missing 85% of the population living in rural areas.[118] Geographical barriers to access may be particularly acute for those from ethnic minority groups.[119] In addition, rural health workers may have little training in the treatment and care of people living with HIV/AIDS.[120]

As a result, people living with HIV/AIDS in rural communities often have lower access to care and support than people living in urban areas. For example, in Cambodia, roughly 8.1% of women in urban areas (aged 15–49 years) had been tested for HIV as compared with 1.6% in rural areas.[121] Among men aged 15–54 years in the Philippines, 4.9% in urban areas and 2.1% in rural areas had been tested for HIV.[122]

At the beginning of the HIV/AIDS epidemic, the vast majority of infected persons were found in urban areas. As a result, HIV prevention, care and treatment services developed mainly in urban areas. Today, however, the situation is changing. As people become ill with opportunistic infections and can no longer work, they often return to their extended families in rural communities for care. This shift is putting additional strain on meagre rural health services and enormous strain on rural family members, who are often poorer and have less access to adequate health services than their urban counterparts.

Although access to treatment for HIV/AIDS has increased greatly over the last few years, in many countries, treatment facilities are largely restricted to urban areas, leaving rural communities underserved. People in rural areas who need treatment must travel long distances to reach treatment facilities. Because of where they live, they must endure high costs for transportation as well as higher opportunity costs associated with lost income. Periods away from home may be particularly difficult for women, who tend to have multiple household responsibilities, including child care.

Economic costs

The economic costs of treatment and care may be broken down into direct costs (medication, user fees), indirect costs (transportation) and opportunity costs (lower productivity and time away from work). The economic costs of treatment and care for HIV/AIDS, including palliative care, treatment for opportunistic infections and ART, often place treatment and care beyond the reach of poor households. Even when the price of treatment and care is relatively low, these costs—as a proportion of household income—are often more than a poor household can bear.

The negative impact of user fees on access by poor households to treatment and care for HIV/AIDS has been substantiated by a number of studies. A meta-analysis of 10 studies found that free treatment was associated with a 29%–31% increase in viral load suppression, compared to treatment paid for by users.[123] Even when sliding fee scales are used, evidence strongly suggests that cost recovery at the point of service delivery hinders the access of many poor households to treatment and care for HIV/AIDS and reduces long-term adherence to treatment.

While ARVs are increasingly being offered free of charge in many countries, the costs associated with seeking care continue to burden many poor families in the Region. For example, in the Philippines, one tablet of Azithromycin, an antibiotic used to treat some opportunistic infections, costs 225 pesos (US$ 4.61).[124] A study found that the average price charged by drug sellers for STI drugs in Hanoi, Viet Nam, was US$ 3.30, ranging from US$ 11.60 to US$ 0.20, with an average of US$ 3.3.[125] Thus, as with access to ART, the financial costs of seeking care for opportunistic infections is likely to reduce the access of men and women, boys and girls in poor communities to adequate health services.

The indirect costs of HIV/AIDS include the provision of nourishing food for the sick family member and/or additional food and schooling expenses for orphans that join the extended family. Transportation to health care facilities can be unaffordable for poor households, particularly if located in rural areas.

Sociocultural barriers

Access to adequate treatment and care for people living with HIV (PLWH) may be limited by the attitudes of health service providers. For example, a study among health professionals in Yunnan Province, China, revealed that 30% of respondents would not treat an HIV-positive individual.[126] Such attitudes among health care providers may deter people from being tested for HIV. Stigma and discrimination have been identified as major factors that prevent men and women from seeking care for HIV/AIDS.[127] A study in China noted that fear of discrimination influenced the use of HIV-related prevention and care services.[128] For people with HIV who require care, discrimination and stigma may force them to seek medical attention repeatedly, thereby delaying care and hence increasing the cost of care, or may deter them from seeking care at all.

Stigma and discrimination may directly or indirectly influence entitlements to ART. For example, it is reported that in Africa, older HIV-infected people are often not considered suitable candidates for ARV therapies. However, a recent study suggests that drugs provide similar benefits to older people (aged 50 and above) as to younger patients.[129] In fact, this study revealed that older patients were more likely to have their HIV blood levels under control, perhaps because they took medications as prescribed.

Inadequate quality of treatment and care

In areas where health services are accessible in terms of distance or affordability, they may not effectively respond to the needs of poor patients. Evidence from many countries shows that the (perceived or actual) quality of health care tends to be substandard, particularly in health facilities located in underserved areas.[130] Many health facilities are neglected or dilapidated, lack supplies and equipment and experience a shortage of essential medicines. For example, the Government of Cambodia recognizes that decades of civil war have left health centres in a dismal state, often lacking electricity and essential medicines and other essential products.[131] In Mongolia, doctors in rural areas often lack essential supplies, such as transportation and medicines.[132] In Solomon Islands, villages near urban centres or along accessible coastal areas enjoy better-quality health services than villages in the remote interior or on isolated stretches of coast.[133]

Health services likewise may be characterized by long waiting times, inconvenient hours, rude and disrespectful staff, and an overall low quality of care.[134] The generally low remuneration and poor working conditions for health staff in underserved areas can result in poor-quality services, absenteeism and many vacancies. In Mongolia, for example, rural doctors benefit less from in-service training than their urban counterparts.[135] Absentee rates among public facility health workers reached 19% in Papua New Guinea.[136] There is some evidence that health service providers are not sufficiently aware or sensitive to the needs and preferences of the poor.[137]

Evidence is lacking on the quality of care for HIV diagnosis, treatment and care in the Region. Evidence from a study in South Africa suggested that poor people are more likely than those who are better-off to seek a diagnosis for HIV at a public facility. The generally low quality of care at public facilities compels better-off people to seek a diagnosis from private providers.[138] In many instances, the poor quality of services requires that poor individuals make repeated visits to multiple health providers.

Clinics providing treatment for STIs in Papua New Guinea are generally found in the larger cities, such as the provincial capitals. In rural health centres, health staff often do not have the training to provide adequate treatment and care for STIs and the appropriate drugs are not always available.[139] In addition, a study found that health staff in Papua New Guinea may not be equipped to manage the effects of ART, including toxicity and possible side-effects.[140] A study of STI treatment practices by drug sellers in Hanoi, Viet Nam, found that none of the drugs sellers visited by simulated clients dispensed treatment for STIs in accordance with national guidelines. In addition, none of the drug sellers provided an adequate daily dose of drugs.[141] In China, it was found that much of the total cost of seeking care may go to unnecessary or inappropriate drugs.[142]

Adherence to treatment

Adherence to ART is well recognized as an essential component of individual and programmatic treatment success.[143] The little evidence available on why some people do not adhere to treatment points to patient- and treatment-related constraints, such as substance abuse, complexity of pill regime and 'pill burden', dietary restrictions and the side-effects of treatment. Corresponding to these constraints, experience shows that adherence to treatment improves when patients are educated prior to beginning treatment, drug regimes are simplified and health staff, family and community members continually support the patient's adherence to treatment.

Research from developed countries documents generally high levels of adherence to treatment. The scant research in developing countries on reasons for non-adherence to treatment by some people suggests that the factors influencing adherence to treatment in developed countries and more affluent communities, such as those outlined above, may not be as relevant in developing countries. Studies carried out from May to September 2005 in Botswana, Tanzania, and Uganda found that, even when ARVs are provided free of charge, the indirect and opportunity costs associated with adherence, including transportation, registration and user fees and wages lost arising from long waiting times at clinics, undermined the motivation of PLWH to adhere to treatment. Hunger during the initial stages of treatment, when the body regains lost strength, was likewise shown to pose difficulties for poor patients who could not afford to increase their food consumption. In addition, some ARVs must be taken with food. PLWH who can afford to eat only once a day are thus unable to adhere to the treatment regime. Not adhering to treatment was similarly linked with inadequate social support, which was found to arise when PLWH did not disclose their status due to stigma or out of fear of discrimination.[144] Similar results were reported by a study of among men and women receiving primary care for HIV in Chennai, India. Among the study population, which was predominantly men aged 31–40 years of age, the financial costs of ART, including the costs of food and travel, were identified as the most significant barriers to adherence. In response, various strategies to cover the costs of ART were documented, including selling property and jewellery, borrowing money from friends and family, and ceasing treatment. Stigma was noted as a key barrier to adherence and, conversely, social support was identified as facilitating treatment.[145] Adherence is critically important for maintaining improved health as well as avoiding the especially difficult problem of drug resistance.

HIV/AIDS may cause or contribute to poverty

The evidence on how HIV/AIDS causes or deepens poverty remains partial, particularly since the epidemic has a shorter history in the Region than in many African countries.[146] Case studies from countries around the world have demonstrated the negative impact of HIV-related illness and death on household income and ability to cope in the short and longer-term. Social networks and coping mechanisms may be strained by the burden of AIDS-related illness and mortality and eroded by discrimination and stigma.[147] Over time, the negative impact that HIV/AIDS appears to have at the household level will probably adversely affect economic development, as adults in their prime are struck down, household investments in children are reduced, human capital falls, and economic returns to business and infrastructure developments drop, among other factors.[148] In African countries, annual economic growth is estimated to have slowed several percentage points because of HIV/AIDS.[149]

The economic impact of HIV/AIDS is evident when resources are diverted to uses that would not have been necessary in the absence of HIV/AIDS, as well as decreased productivity due to the disease.[150] AIDS can contribute to poverty through a number of routes: a reduction or loss in income arising from lower productivity or lost work; the catastrophic costs of care; an increased dependency ratio (increased number of family members depending on fewer individuals earning an income); loss of human and social capital among communities and the country as a whole (effects on the social structure of local communities; the erosion of existing social networks and traditional mechanisms of support); and the reduced national income of a country.[151] The impact of AIDS on households and communities is particularly severe when it affects the economically active population. Figure 9 presents a flow chart on how HIV/AIDS induces and deepens poverty.

Catastrophic costs of care

In the world's poorest countries (where the HIV epidemic is the most profound), many people, particularly the poor, have to pay for health care from their own pockets.[152] A study of health care seeking in Cote d'Ivoire, Tanzania and Thailand observed that people who died of AIDS-related causes had more likely sought medical care and incurred out-of-pocket medical expenses than people who died of other illnesses. Household expenditures were also much higher in households with someone suffering from AIDS than other medical causes.[153] The cost of care for HIV/AIDS in Thailand was estimated to be US$ 835 per person in 1992 and US$ 1335 in 2002.[154]

Families may thus make great sacrifices to provide treatment, relief and comfort for sick relatives. In a Thai study, families spent an average of US$ 1000 during the last year of life of a person with AIDS, the equivalent of an average annual income.[155] Caring for a person with HIV/AIDS can drain a family's economic resources, resulting in poverty and, in many cases, destitution.[156] Finally, the costs of funerals are high. With rising death rates in many developing countries, the financial burden of funerals can contribute to family poverty.

The opportunity costs of caring for a family member with HIV/AIDS are great. First, the family loses the wages of the caregiver, usually a woman, who leaves employment to care for the sick family member. Second, less time is devoted to income-generating activities within the home such as farming, tending to animals, or producing handicrafts. And third, young people, whether infected or caregivers, may lose opportunities for further schooling and job training. The annual lifetime earnings lost to an AIDS death was estimated to amount to 11 times the annual cost

Figure 9: HIV/AIDS can induce and deepen poverty

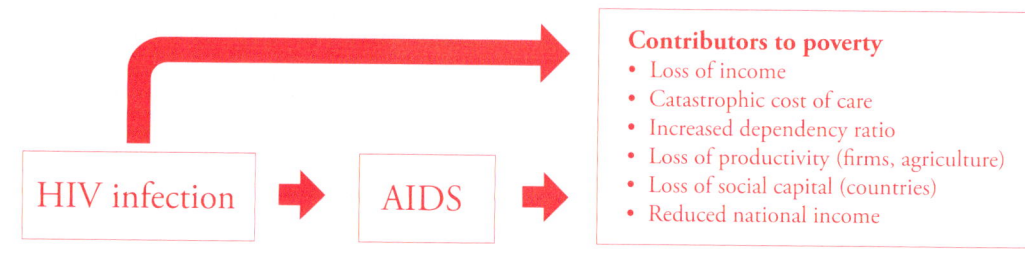

Source: Adeyi *et al.* 2001.

of treatment in Sri Lanka. In Nepal, these costs were equivalent to more than four times the per capita annual income.[157]

In many parts of the world, when people with HIV begin to experience the debilitating effects of severe opportunistic infections, they return to their native or parents' homes for care, treatment and support. A study of the impact of HIV/AIDS on older people in Cambodia and Thailand found that parents were commonly involved in caring for their fatally ill children. Such caring occurred through both living and care-giving arrangements. Among the study population, roughly 50% of Cambodian parents reported reduced economic activities as a result of their children being sick with AIDS.[158]

Young adults who return home with AIDS often bring their children with them. As a result, older parents are suddenly burdened with the care not only of their sick children, but also of their grandchildren. These grandchildren eventually become orphans, increasing the dependency ratio. The stress of trying to address the needs of additional family members poses both a financial and an emotional burden on older adults.

Loss of productivity and reduced household income

A vicious cycle results from HIV: the epidemic reduces economic growth and increases poverty, which then fuels the epidemic. The vast majority of PLWH are between the ages of 15 and 49, and in the prime of their working lives. AIDS weakens economic activity by squeezing productivity, adding costs, diverting productive resources, and depleting skills. For example, managers in one sugar estate in Kenya noted increased absenteeism (8000 days of work lost due to sickness between 1995 and 1997), lower productivity (a 50% drop in processing), and higher overtime costs (healthy workers had to work overtime when colleagues were sick). The same company reported that the costs of social benefits for health care and funeral costs related to HIV infection have risen sharply.[159]

Absenteeism also means a loss of skilled labour. Businesses have to train new workers for skilled jobs, only to have them become sick and leave their employment. In the United States of America, companies with around 1000 employees reported that the five-year cost to their business ranged from US$ 17 000 to US$ 32 000 for each worker with HIV/AIDS. Thus, supporting prevention programmes makes good economic sense for employers.[160]

The loss of a prime-age adult to severe illness and death likely has long-term implications for household well-being. In a study of households with a member sick with AIDS or a member who had recently died of AIDS in South Africa, 60% of households surveyed reported lost income as a consequence of HIV/AIDS and 22% of children under the age of 15 years reported having lost a parent.[161] A second study analysed data from the Kagera Region of Tanzania to estimate the long-term implications of adult death in households in a rural area with a high prevalence of HIV. The results suggest that adult mortality, especially of women, has a significant negative impact upon the welfare of surviving household members, as measured in household consumption. Within five years of the adult death, household consumption decreased by 7% on average. This negative effect appeared to lessen with time, as no significant impact on household consumption was observed six to 13 years after the death of the prime-age adult.[162] In Thailand, roughly 60% of households surveyed had spent all their savings to help a household member living with AIDS and 19% had sold their assets.[163] Studies from East Asia explained that catastrophic illness, including TB, HIV and severe malaria, triggered 50% of financial crises in poor families.[164] Household surveys show that families living with HIV/AIDS in Asia and Africa experienced a 40%–60% reduction in income.[165]

Evidence from sub-Saharan Africa reveals that, as the epidemic progresses, AIDS can result in the loss of farming skills, the decline of agricultural services, the gradual disappearance of the productive capacity to work the land and the disintegration of rural livelihoods. In the last two decades, AIDS has killed seven million agricultural workers in Africa alone. As a result, thousands of farming communities have been devastated, leaving families struggling to produce enough food to survive.[166] While the impact of HIV/AIDS on livelihoods in the Region has not been substantiated, it may emerge as an important issue in the future. This is because, in many countries in the Region, the population is predominantly rural and thus the spread of HIV/AIDS interacts dynamically with rural livelihoods, which are largely agriculture based.[167]

HIV-related stigma and discrimination leading to poverty

HIV/AIDS-related discrimination and stigma may lead to increased poverty among PLWH and their households through a number of unique pathways. Most directly, stigma and discrimination can lead to job loss or abandonment of PLWH and their immediate relatives.

Although international human rights law prohibits discrimination against PLWH, or those perceived to be at higher risk of infection, the reality is that these people are more likely to lose a job or be denied employment. Despite the fact that HIV is not readily transmitted in the majority of workplace settings, the supposed risk of transmission has been used by numerous employers to terminate or refuse employment. Pre-employment screening takes place in many industries, particularly where health benefits are available to employees. Employer-sponsored health insurance programmes have come under increasing financial pressure in countries that have been seriously affected by HIV/AIDS. Some employers have used this pressure to deny employment to PLWH. Businesses face enormous challenges in responding to AIDS. Sometimes, when PLWH are open about their sero-status at work, they are likely to experience stigmatization, ostracism and job loss.[168] Thus, HIV/AIDS reduces access to employment and contributes to poverty.

Some evidence suggests that children with HIV/AIDS or children with HIV-positive parents may experience discrimination, with negative repercussions in the long term. In India, children with HIV or whose parents are infected with HIV may be expelled from or segregated at school. Orphanages and other residential institutions may likewise not admit children who are HIV-positive and these children may be denied medical care.[169] Such discrimination may reduce their opportunity to gain an education and or obtain adequate health care.

Poverty impact of HIV/AIDS through education

AIDS threatens the educational system and, therefore, undermines the human capital of a country. A decline in school enrolment is one of the most visible effects of the epidemic. The reasons for this decline include removal of children for care-giving activities; the inability of families to pay for school fees, books and uniforms; AIDS-related infertility and decline in the birth rate; and children becoming infected with HIV/AIDS.

Many children must leave school to care for sick family members or orphaned siblings, thus jeopardizing their education and future employment opportunities. Studies from Uganda show that, following the death of one or both parents, the probability of an orphan going to school is halved and those who do go to school spend less time there than they formerly did.[170] A case study from southwest China found that orphans and older children with HIV-infected parents were less likely to be in school than their peers.[171] Many orphaned children assume responsibilities as the head of the household and undoubtedly face great economic difficulties. When orphaned children are cared for by others, the caring family's limited resources must stretch to accommodate the additional needs of these children.[172] A study of youth who had lost one or both parents to AIDS in Thailand noted that although these youth were cared for by their extended families, their households tended to suffer from financial hardship.[173] In addition, orphaned children may be denied their inheritance. Therefore, the cycle of poverty, poor education, and vulnerability to risk-taking continues as these young people negotiate life with little financial or emotional support. Thus, the risk of contracting HIV/AIDS becomes a very real concern.

Impact of HIV/AIDS on younger people

An estimated 15 million children have been orphaned as a result of the death of their parents from AIDS. Roughly 12 million of these children live in sub-Saharan Africa.[174] Although data in this regard are scarce in the Region, the number of children orphaned due to AIDS will likely rise as the epidemic progresses. An estimated 22 000 children were orphaned by AIDS in Viet Nam in 2001.[175]

The HIV/AIDS epidemic affects children and young people in the following ways:
- disintegration of traditional support structures and social safety nets;
- reduced survival and development rates of children through its impact on health, family livelihoods, social welfare and protection;
- discrimination and exclusion from the community as a result of stigmatization;
- loss of quality education due to the loss of school teachers to AIDS; and
- reduced opportunities for education due to exclusion or the need to redirect household spending towards medical treatment, which severely limits funds for schooling.[176]

Impact of HIV/AIDS on older people

The impact of HIV/AIDS on older people is rarely considered. While some are infected with HIV, a far greater number are affected by the infection of significant others, especially their adult children and orphaned grandchildren. The effects on older people include:
- the added burden of family care-giving
- providing financial and material support to family members
- raising surviving grandchildren
- suffering emotional stress
- losing the financial support that their child would normally have provided.

The effect of HIV on national income

HIV/AIDS prevents people from contributing to economic growth and thus increases poverty. Only recently has HIV/AIDS been recognized as a major development issue.[177]

The increase in HIV/AIDS morbidity and mortality affects economic and social development.[178] In many countries, the cumulative effects of the epidemic could have catastrophic consequences for long-term economic growth and seriously damage the prospects for poverty reduction. Until recently, most experts believed that a generalized HIV/AIDS epidemic at 10% adult prevalence would reduce economic growth by about 0.5% per year.[179] A range of studies point to the negative net effect of the epidemic on per capita gross domestic product (GDP) growth, and in some instances, AIDS is responsible for a substantial decline. Countries with 20% adult prevalence rates estimate a drop in GDP growth of 2.6%. Calculations in sub-Saharan Africa suggest that the rate of economic growth has fallen by as much as 4% as a result of AIDS.[180] Thus, AIDS is contributing to the deepening of poverty in many resource-poor countries.

Although the economic impact of HIV/AIDS is known in part, the full economic impact on women has not been quantified. This is because their work in the home, the community and in productive work outside the formal sector has not been adequately documented.[181]

The links between gender and HIV/AIDS

Gender roles and relations have a significant influence on the course and impact of the HIV/AIDS epidemic. Women's subordinate position relative to men places them at considerable disadvantage with respect to their access to resources and goods, decision-making power, choices, and opportunities across all spheres of life. Gender roles influence the ways that men and women are vulnerable to HIV transmission and mediate the impact of living with HIV/AIDS. Gender relations are in turn affected by social, cultural and economic factors and can determine the differential access of men and women to care and support services.[182]

Almost as many women as men are now dying of AIDS, as the gap in HIV prevalence rates among men and women is narrowing. Globally, 15.4 million women were living with HIV/AIDS in 2007, 1.6 million more than the 13.8 million in 2001.[183] Since 2002, the number of women living with HIV increased in every region. East Asia experienced the sharpest increase, with 56% in two years, followed by Eastern Europe and Central Asia with 48%.[184] In 2006, women constituted 29% of adults living with HIV/AIDS in Asia and 47% in the Pacific. Figure 10 presents the proportion of adults living with HIV who are women in all regions from 1990 to 2007.

Equally alarmingly, young women are becoming infected at younger ages than men, and are estimated to comprise 67% of all newly infected 15- to 24-year-olds in developing countries.[185] Over 75% of HIV infections are transmitted through sexual relations between men and women.[186] In countries where young people account for the high proportion of all new infections, HIV-positive women may outnumber men by as much as six times.[187] Therefore, addressing gender roles and power dynamics between women and men, and how they impact on sexual relations and decision-making, is essential for effectively halting and ultimately reversing the epidemic.

Vulnerability of women and girls to HIV/AIDS

Women's biological vulnerability to HIV/AIDS

Research shows that the risk of becoming infected with HIV during unprotected vaginal intercourse is as much as two to four times higher for women than men.[188] Male-to-female transmission is more efficient during vaginal intercourse because women have a larger surface area of mucosa exposed to their partner's semen. Semen has a higher concentration of HIV than a woman's vaginal secretions. In addition, women are also vulnerable to other STIs, which can multiply the risk of contracting HIV by as much as tenfold.[189] Younger women are even more at risk because their immature cervix and scant vaginal secretions make them prone to vaginal mucosal lacerations. There is also evidence that women become more vulnerable to HIV infection after menopause. In addition, tearing and bleeding during intercourse, whether from rough sex, rape or prior genital mutilation, multiply the risk of HIV infection. Anal intercourse is sometimes preferred to vaginal intercourse because it is thought to preserve

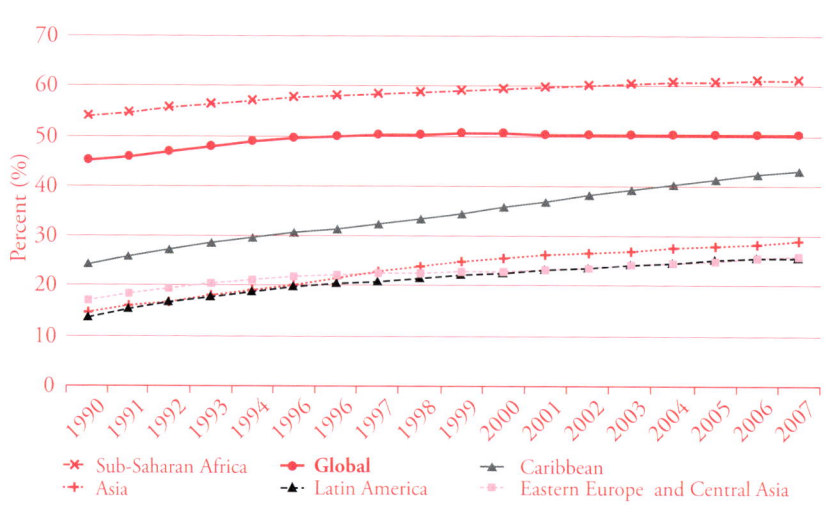

Figure 10: Percentage of adults (15+) living with HIV who are female, 1990–2007

Source: Joint United Nations Programme on HIV/AIDS 2007g.

virginity and avoid the risk of pregnancy. However, anal intercourse often tears the delicate anal tissues and provides easy access for the virus.[190]

Mother-to-child transmission (MTCT) of HIV is a key mode of HIV infection in children. An estimated 420 000 children are infected each year, 90% through MTCT. Without preventive treatment, up to 40% of children born to HIV-positive women will be infected. Of those who are infected, it is believed that about two thirds are infected during pregnancy, mostly around the time of delivery, and about one third are infected through breast-feeding. Therefore, prevention of MTCT is a major health need.

Gender norms and the sociocultural vulnerability of women and girls

Gender norms within societies influence the attitudes, assumptions and behaviours that are prescribed for men and women, boys and girls. Gender norms tend to be underpinned by unequal power relations that result in women's weaker bargaining position relative to the men within their households and wider communities. In this way, gender norms can restrict the ability of women to negotiate safer sexual practices with their partners, placing even women who remain faithful to one partner at increased risk of HIV infection.

Sociocultural norms, beliefs and customs can have a direct effect on vulnerability to HIV infection. Girls and women are often raised to be submissive and unaware of sexual matters until marriage. They often fear reprisals from their partners and others, or being identified as promiscuous, immodest or unfaithful, if they raise issues related to sexuality, and sexual health, including STI/HIV prevention. Also, while many women suffering from STI are asymptomatic, when they do experience subsequent STI-related problems, they tend to accept them as normal.

Early marriage and vulnerability associated with age and cultural norms may promote respect of men's authority in sexual matters and contraceptive use, and dictate sex as a wife's duty, regardless of her preferences or the risks to herself. Thus marriage can be a major risk factor for women who are powerless to negotiate condom use or influence their husband's extramarital behaviour. It is estimated that 60%–80% of HIV-positive African women have had sexual intercourse solely with their husbands.[191] An estimated 50% of new infections in Cambodia are transmitted sexually from husbands to wives.[192]

Typically, women are expected to leave the initiative and decision-making about sex to men, whose needs and demands are expected to dominate. A double standard often operates, whereby women may be blamed or evicted for infidelity (real or suspected), while men are expected or allowed to have multiple partners. In addition, women from traditional families may be under intense familial pressure to produce children while being unable to admit that they have contracted HIV from a husband who is unfaithful.

In many societies, the high social value placed on virginity may pressure parents and the community to ensure that young women are kept ignorant about sexual matters. This prevents them from seeking information about sex or services related to sexual health.[193] Sexual cleansing is a custom based on the belief that a man can be cured of HIV/AIDS if he has sex with a young virgin. Although more prevalent in Africa, there is some evidence that this custom extends into the Western Pacific Region. In Cambodia, the fear of AIDS may have increased the demand for virgins. The belief that having sex with a virgin will cure a man of AIDS has also been attributed in one study as driving the demand for virgin sex workers and increasing rape among young virgin girls in Cambodia.[194]

The vulnerability of women and girls is further compounded by the following factors:

- **Lack of education and awareness.** Women and girls typically achieve lower rates of education that men and boys. Besides, millions of young girls are brought up with little knowledge of their reproductive system or how HIV and STI are transmitted and prevented.[195] For example, one study found that girls in the 15–19 year old age group in Ethiopia, Malawi, Tanzania, Zambia and Zimbabwe were found to be five to six times more likely to become infected than boys, through lack of knowledge.[196]

- **Lack of economic opportunities**. Failure to ensure the human rights of women to equal access to education and employment opportunities reinforces their economic dependence. This reliance may be placed on a husband or partner, a few steady male partners who have fathered their children, or for women in prostitution, a succession of clients. Such reliance on a partner may reduce the ability of a woman to protect herself from HIV infection, such as negotiating the use of a condom or leaving a partner who is engaging in high-risk sexual activity.

- **Lack of access to services**. Access to services and treatment are unavailable or unaffordable for a significant portion of HIV-infected women, particularly those living in developing countries.[197] The results are tragic. For example, in Botswana and South Africa, it is estimated that one half of today's 15-year-olds will die of AIDS.[198] In addition, health service providers are often unsympathetic, judgmental, and unprepared to diagnose and treat STIs. Evidence from Africa indicates that men are more likely than women to be admitted to hospital, and family resources are likely to be used (and potentially depleted) for medications and care for male rather then female members of the household.[199]

- **Conflict and civil unrest**. Migration or displacement as a result of civil strife, natural disasters, drought, famine, and political oppression has a greater impact on women's vulnerability to HIV infection compared to men.[200] About 75% of all refugees and displaced people are women and children.[201] Widespread rape of women has been documented in times of war. Women migrant workers, refugees or returnees are often more vulnerable to some form of sexual barter as they try to negotiate employment, necessary documentation or places to live.[202] In addition, undocumented migrant women experience limited options, have low status, receive low pay and are often isolated in their work (including marriage, domestic, factory and sex work).[203] These situations place women in vulnerable and powerless positions, with little ability to refuse or negotiate safe sex, increasing their risk for HIV/AIDS infection.

- **HIV and female prostitution**. The most powerless and vulnerable people are children and women coerced into the sex trade by traffickers, with an estimated 2 million girls aged five to 15 being coerced into the trade each year. Prostitution is often the only means of financial security for women; however, they may not have the power to negotiate condom use or to protect themselves from HIV. Sex workers may risk violence or loss of income if they request the use of condoms. However, in some brothels, sex workers have banded together to insist on their use.[204]

- **Stigma and discrimination**. The stigma of HIV/AIDS is highly complex, dynamic and deeply ingrained in society. It is linked to broader, existing inequalities and to society's often negative view of expressions of sexuality.[205] Women are often blamed for the spread of HIV, even though the majority have been infected by their partner. Stigma and discrimination in relation to HIV and STI are much greater for women than for men. Women who face stigma risk violence, abandonment, neglect, destitution and ostracism from family and the community. Stigma also deters women from seeking care and treatment services.[206]

- **Gender-based violence**. Gender-based violence encompasses physical, sexual and psychological violence. While both men and women may experience gender-based violence, women and children comprise the overwhelming majority of those affected. Globally, violence against women is most common in the private sphere and is usually carried out by an intimate male partner, family member or acquaintance. The lifetime prevalence of physical or sexual violence, or both, among women ranges from 15% to 71%. A high incidence of non-consensual sex, particularly among young women, has been reported.[207] It is increasingly apparent that gender-based violence is an important risk factor for HIV/AIDS. Studies from Rwanda, Tanzania and South Africa estimate that the risk of HIV was three times greater for women who had experienced violence than for women who had not.[208]

Gender-based violence, particularly forced or coerced sex, enhances the biological vulnerability of women (and men) to HIV infection. While the risk of HIV infection varies with the type of sexual exposure (vaginal, anal or oral), the likelihood of infection rises with the degree of trauma, vaginal lacerations and abrasions. The risks of transmission associated with forced or coerced sex tend to be higher among young women and girls because their vaginal tracts are immature and may tear easily. Gender-based violence has been associated with increased risk of STIs, which are a risk factor for HIV infection. Conversely, a study among men in India found that men with STIs were 2.5 times more likely to abuse their wives than men without STIs.[209]

When women experience violence, they are more likely to engage in behaviour that increases their risk of HIV infection, such as engaging with multiple partners and transactional sex. A population-based survey found that among all the sites surveyed, except for in Ethiopia, women who had experienced intimate partner violence were more likely to know that their partners were having sexual relations with other women, than women who had not experienced intimate partner violence.[210] Violence or the threat of violence may also reduce the ability of women to negotiate condom use, access information on HIV/AIDS and seek prevention, treatment and care for HIV/AIDS.

The role of girls and women in family care-giving and orphan care

When a family member with HIV/AIDS becomes ill, the vast majority of home-based caregivers are women and girls. This may lead to considerable hardship for women and girls.[211] Older women become isolated, exhausted, overwhelmed with their care-giving responsibilities, and in some cases, they may be unable to cope. When young girls become responsible for the care of a sick family member, they may have to leave school and quit other age-appropriate activities. They lose opportunities for education, job training, or learning about income-generating activities. They may also become isolated from friends and often become depressed. Both women and young girls may lack education on caring for a family member with HIV/AIDS. They may know little about universal precautions or basic nursing care. When the person with AIDS dies, the extended family (again, most often women and girls) must assume responsibilities for orphan care. Box 3 provides an example of the stress placed on women as family caregivers.

Gender bias in HIV/AIDS prevention, treatment and research

In many countries in the Region, the quality of care provided by health staff working in poor and marginalized communities tends to be inadequate. Often, such poor quality care encompasses discriminatory attitudes towards women who seek prevention, diagnosis, treatment and care for HIV/AIDS. In some developing countries, HIV-positive women are likely to be treated very differently from men, once they seek care.[212]

> **Box 3: Experiences of women as family caregivers in Botswana**
>
> A 34-year-old woman is caring for her sister and her sister's child, both of whom have AIDS and tuberculosis as a co-infection. Seven younger sisters and brothers and 15 children are also living in the caregiver's home (12 of these children belong to her and to her brothers and sisters; three are orphans from a deceased brother and sister-in-law, both of whom died of AIDS). The caregiver's parents died five years ago. The caregiver has no formal education, and the family survives on a destitute allowance. She makes a pittance buying chicken in bulk and selling pieces. She also sells a local beer. The caregiver describes both the sister and her child as "very ill and getting worse". Both patients have productive coughs, and the sister complains of dizziness and headaches. The infected sister has bouts of crying, after which she says she feels better. The infected baby was hospitalized with a fractured leg three months ago. Upon discharge, the child was prescribed a rich protein supplement and additional milk. Because the family cannot not afford the supplements, the child must eat a light porridge made with water. The caregiver has to wash her sister, help her dress and help her go to the toilet. The baby needs total care. In addition, the caregiver and one of her younger sisters manages the home; they collect water from a communal standpipe, collect firewood, cook, shop and do the daily tasks of the household. She explains her responsibilities:
>
> *"I take care of all my younger sisters and brothers and I am responsible for the schoolwork. I am the one who is responsible for all the orphans. I make sure [my sister and her child] have enough blankets and I heat the water and bathe them each day. My heart is always painful because of taking care of the baby and the mother. I do feel pains to such a point that my heart beats faster, and I do feel like crying. I don't know if there is any help I can receive because I am always thinking alone and not understanding what is happening."*
>
> Source: World Health Organization 2000e.

Health workers have been found to be disrespectful and judgemental of women who seek prevention, diagnosis, treatment and care for HIV/AIDS. Evidence suggests that health workers do not always seek the informed consent of women before testing them for HIV.[213] The results of HIV diagnosis do not always remain confidential and are instead shared with male partners or in-laws. For example, a study carried out in Mumbai found that when women were diagnosed with HIV, health workers disclosed their status to husbands based on the notion that the women themselves could not understand the diagnosis.[214]

Once diagnosed with HIV, women may be denied services by health workers or coerced into accepting services that are inadequately explained. Men are more likely to be "excused" by health staff for their behaviours that result in HIV infection, whereas women are not.[215] A study in Nepal observed that the fear of infection prompted health care providers to refuse treatment to HIV-positive women.[216]

Health workers have been found to discriminate against HIV-positive women, particularly with regards to reproduction and pregnancy. A study in India and Thailand observed that many HIV-positive women experienced limited reproductive health choices and that decisions were predominantly made by health workers, husbands or in-laws.[217] Another study of HIV-positive people in India, Indonesia, the Philippines and Thailand carried out in 2001-2002 reported that, upon receiving diagnosis of their HIV-positive status, an estimated 45% of women were advised by health workers to not have children, while only 18% of HIV-positive men received the same advice. In addition, 12% of the women surveyed were coerced into having an abortion or sterilization.[218]

Research shows that vaginal microbicides can make a very substantial difference by widening people's choice of protective interventions.[219] However, the microbicide concept has only recently received sufficient support to allow progress to be made. Pharmaceutical companies have not so far regarded microbicides as providing economic incentives for substantial investment; however, nongovernmental organizations (NGOs) and other bodies are now giving serious consideration to the matter.

Prevention messages of 100% condom use for sex workers may put them at risk of abuse from their clients.[220] In addition, female condoms have not received the social marketing campaigns that were applied to the sale and use of male condoms. Female condoms are more expensive and are rarely subsidized by governments. As a result, few women know of, or can afford female condoms that would provide them with a measure of control in the prevention of HIV transmission.

Despite women being diagnosed with HIV/AIDS from the early 1980s, research has often been gender-biased. At the end of 1999, women accounted for only 12% of total trial participants (usually for mother-to-child transmission). Little research has been done to investigate the differences between men and women in disease progression, opportunistic infections and management, despite apparent differences in length of survival, levels of viral load and drug toxicity. For example, recent evidence suggests that although men and women appear to progress from HIV to AIDS at the same rate, women appear to progress to AIDS with lower viral load levels than men.[221] If viral load was considered in the criteria for treatment initiation, instead of CD4 cell count, which is the current practice, women's access to effective treatment could be delayed.[222] In addition, the sero-markers to determine when to start ARV therapy were developed for men. Therefore, ARV treatment and the management of opportunistic infections may need to be tailored for women and men differently.[223] Ignoring the differences in disease progression for men and women can lead to gender-biased conclusions and solutions.

Gender bias in the law

Laws regarding marriage, divorce and child custody that are discriminatory can impede women's ability to seek protection or to leave relationships in which they or their children are exposed to the risk of HIV infection. In some settings, women have no legal right to refuse sex with their husbands.[224] In Cambodia, for example, a study documented the widely held belief that husbands have a right to the bodies of their wives.[225] In other areas, the laws regarding marriage and divorce have different implications for men and women. For example, Philippine law defines extramarital affairs differently for men than for women.[226] Under such circumstances, women find it difficult to assert their preference for safer sex, for their partner's fidelity or for no sex at all.

Where appropriate laws and policies are in place, they may remain ineffective unless women are aware of and able to exercise their rights. Moreover, concern is repeatedly raised about the lack of political will among governments to put gender-sensitive policies into practice. Research conducted among 500 sex workers reported that 56% of respondents believed that the criminalization of their work played a role in the spread of HIV. This study also reported that 84% of sex workers were forced into unprotected sex by clients and that they had no legal recourse in the event of rape and abuse. In fact, the report noted that sex workers believed that the law itself undermined efforts to design and implement effective interventions among prostitutes.[227]

Gender and the vulnerability of men and boys to HIV/AIDS

The ways in which gender norms influence the vulnerability of men, and especially young boys, to HIV/AIDS is beginning to be increasingly recognized. Social norms reinforce their lack of understanding of sexual health issues and at the same time celebrate promiscuity. Throughout the world, "masculinity" is often associated with the "male drive", physical strength, power and negative behaviours such as violence and sexual risk-taking. For example, in Cambodia, notions of masculinity are associated with multiple sex partners and frequent sex.[228] However, it is important to recognize that such forms of "masculinity" oppress both men and women. For example, men who do not conform to the "male" stereotype are often ostracized and ridiculed as effeminate.[229] At the same time, these norms place women in positions of weaker power and thus at higher risk. Therefore, sociocultural gender norms also contribute substantially to men's vulnerability in the following ways:

- **Risk-taking behaviours**. Factors such as age, education, income, self-esteem and peer relations influence the risk-taking behaviours of men and boys. Risky situations involving sexual and drug-taking behaviour in men are supported by cultural beliefs and expectations about "manhood".[230] Results from sexual behaviour studies around the world indicate that heterosexual men (both single and married), as well as homosexual and bisexual men, have higher reported rates of partner changes than women.[231] Norms related to multiple partners for men are condoned implicitly or explicitly in the majority of societies, but they contribute to a greater risk of HIV. The use of drugs and alcohol has been identified as contributing substantially to men's vulnerability to HIV.[232] Mood-altering drugs (legal and illegal) promote risky behaviour by affecting decision-making abilities. In such circumstances, the use of condoms is less likely, and other behaviours and sexual practices that increase the risk of HIV transmission are more likely to occur.[233, 234]

- **Men who have sex with men**. Sex between men occurs in all countries and societies. However, social and cultural norms and epidemiological categorizations of sexuality can hide the true extent to which it occurs.[235] The fact that sex between men is socially stigmatizing (and in many cases, illegal) contributes to an inability to reach these men with information and services to reduce their risk of STI and HIV infection. Furthermore, research shows that in many societies, many MSM also have sex with women, and that bisexual behaviours are often accompanied by a wide range of sexual identities, homosexuality being only one of them.[236, 237]

- **Lack of access to men-focused services and resources**. Traditionally, family planning and reproductive health services have focused almost exclusively on women. Services such as family planning, voluntary HIV counselling and testing (VCT) and sexual and reproductive health are often unavailable to men.[238] Access to services for male contraception can be difficult for young men and boys.

- **Lack of access to information and education**. One of the most important "gaps" in working for improved sexual health for men is the absence of clear information about men's attitudes towards sex and sexuality. In fact, for men, there is little reliable information on sex.[239] Moreover, men and boys are often expected to be sexually knowledgeable and experienced. Some adults believe that young people, especially young men, are naturally sexually promiscuous and that giving them information about sex will make them more sexually active. This lack of education leads to a perpetuation of sexual stereotypes and encourages risky behaviour. Because sexual ignorance is socially unacceptable, young men are reluctant to admit their lack of knowledge and cannot seek it. They lack knowledge on contraception, male sexuality, safe sex practices and prevention of STIs including HIV.

- **HIV/AIDS in the military and the police**. Throughout the world, military personnel (mostly men) are among the populations most susceptible to HIV/AIDS. Military and peacekeeping missions often involve lengthy periods away from home. As a result, service personnel often look for ways to relieve loneliness, stress and sexual needs. In addition, the militaristic ethos tends to excuse or even encourage risk-taking. Thus, military personnel and camps, including peacekeeping forces, tend to attract sex workers and dealers of illicit drugs.[240] Recently, comparative studies of sexual behaviour in France, the United Kingdom and the United States of America showed that military personnel have a much higher risk of HIV infection than groups of the same age and sex in the civilian population. Armed forces in other parts of the world reflect similar patterns.

Members of the police force are vulnerable to HIV/AIDS because they interact with and exert power over populations considered to be at high risk of HIV/AIDS, such as sex workers and injecting drug users, especially where such behaviour is criminalized. For example, the prevalence of HIV/AIDS is estimated to be 8% among police and military personnel in Cambodia. Various studies suggest that 20%–50% of the Cambodian police force had visited sex workers in the past year.

- **HIV in prisons and closed settings**. The conditions in prisons and closed settings often facilitate the spread of HIV. In many countries, the prevalence of HIV/AIDS in prisons and other detention centres is high, often many times higher than in the general population.[241] The HIV prevalence in prisons was estimated to be 4%–22% in Indonesia and 28.4% in Viet Nam.[242] Research suggests that people entering prisons tend to have a relatively high incidence of HIV/AIDS.[243] This may stem from the fact that certain populations vulnerable to HIV/AIDS also face an increased likelihood of incarceration because of their involvement in sex work and injecting drug use, which are illegal in many countries. The general lack of legal aid suggests that prison populations may be drawn predominantly from poor and marginalized groups. A high proportion of inmates are incarcerated for drug-related crimes and many find ways to continue taking drugs while in prison. In male-only institutions, male inmates may have sex with other men. While sex among male and female prisoners maybe consensual, coerced sex may be common and can be a tool to assert dominance within violent prison settings. Unprotected sex is often rampant. In many cases, prisoners are unable to take measures to protect themselves against HIV/AIDS, or to influence factors such as overcrowding and health and the often substandard nutrition in prisons. Prisoners largely depend on ill-equipped prison authorities for information on HIV/AIDS and access to condoms, clean needles and appropriate health services, including care, treatment and support for HIV/AIDS.[244]

3. Why is it important for health professionals to address poverty and gender concerns in HIV/AIDS?

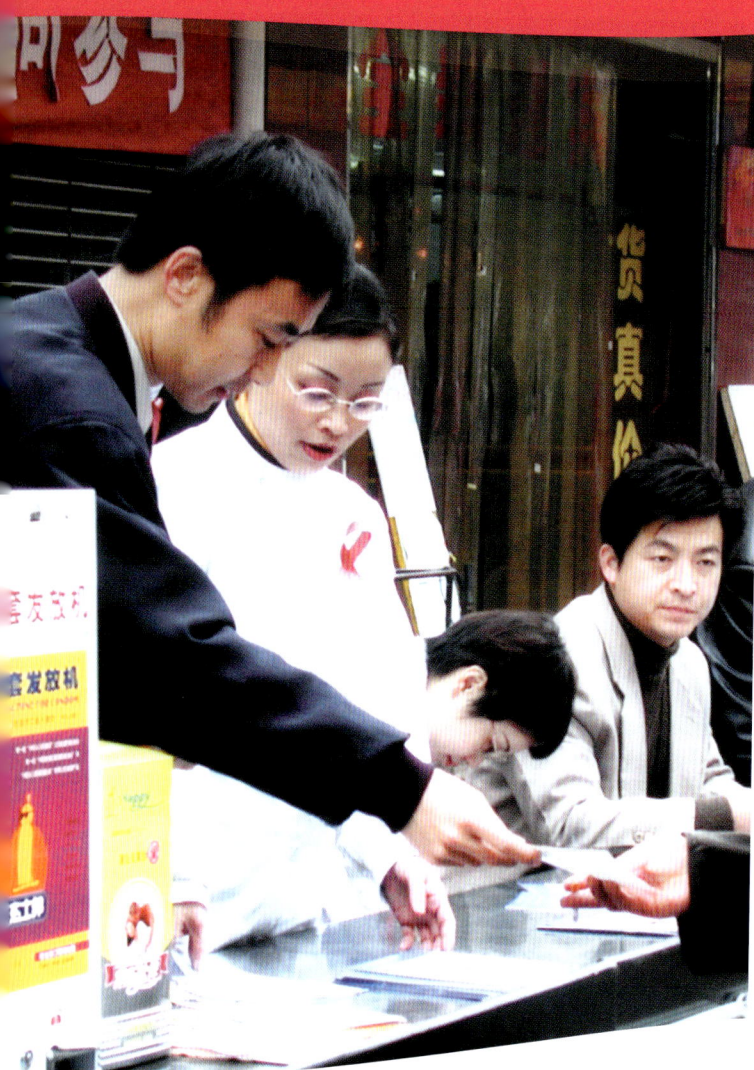

Integrating Poverty and Gender into Health Programmes: *A Sourcebook for Health Professionals*
Module on HIV/AIDS

3. Why is it important for health professionals to address poverty and gender concerns in HIV/AIDS?

Based on the evidence presented in the preceding section, poverty and gender inequality appear to be key factors influencing the spread of HIV/AIDS in the Region. Poverty and gender inequality, both independently and in concert, are associated with increased vulnerability to HIV infection. While the pathways are complex, evidence highlights how poverty and gender inequality limit the ability of poor men and women to protect themselves from HIV, such as by negotiating safe sex and receiving adequate information on HIV/AIDS. The economic and social costs associated with seeking preventive and curative health care for HIV/IDS likewise appear to reduce access of poor men and women to prevention, care and treatment services. With this given, three broad rationales are now considered for giving attention to poverty and gender issues in HIV/AIDS interventions: efficiency, equity, and human rights.

Efficiency

Promising developments in the prevention, treatment and care of HIV/AIDS have taken place throughout the Region. However, the number of people living with HIV continues to grow. In many countries in the Region, HIV is spreading from vulnerable groups to the general population, and the proportion of women with HIV is likewise mounting. As discussed above, vulnerability to HIV infection is often driven by factors related to poverty and gender inequality. Poor and marginalized individuals tend to face considerable constraints when seeking to reduce their exposure to HIV/AIDS; poverty and low education, among other factors, have been associated with an increased likelihood of engaging in risky behaviour. Prevailing gender norms among communities in the Region may likewise hamper the ability of women and men to reduce their exposure to HIV/AIDS. For many women, the largest risk of infection is simply being married. Gender norms among communities in the Region may associate masculinity with violence and frequent sex. Societies, therefore, must address the gender norms and gender relations that underpin such vulnerabilities. Strategies that seek to transform gender relations and empower men and women to protect themselves from HIV offer an efficient means of enhancing the effectiveness of existing preventive measures.

The generally unequal access of poor and marginalized individuals and households to preventive and curative health care services in the Region further suggests that investments in HIV prevention, treatment and care may not be reaching poor populations. Tailoring preventive efforts to meet the needs of poor and marginalized communities can work towards ensuring that these populations benefit from investments in HIV prevention and can strengthen HIV/AIDS prevention and treatment efforts. Similarly, the limited availability and economic costs associated with accessing treatment for AIDS may place ART beyond the reach of many poor individuals. Innovative strategies are thus required to address poverty- and gender-related concerns in HIV/AIDS prevention, treatment and care. Together, these approaches can improve the overall efficiency of prevention, treatment and care for HIV, thereby promoting the achievement of the goals for HIV prevention, treatment and care.

The efficiency gains from improved targeting of poor men and women in HIV/AIDS prevention, treatment and care may be even more significant when attention is drawn to the central role that health improvements among poor populations play in poverty-reduction strategies. The long-term nature of care and treatment for AIDS may impoverish households and force already poor households into deeper poverty. The impact of AIDS may likewise be transmitted across generations, with the rise of AIDS orphans and intergenerational poverty. Efforts to ensure that poor households benefit equitably from prevention, treatment and care for HIV/AIDS can improve the well-being of poor individuals and protect them from the economic and social costs of AIDS-related illness and death. At the national level, such interventions may contribute towards improved economic growth and poverty reduction

Equity

Equity in health may be defined as the "absence of systematic disparities in health (or major social determinants) between groups with different levels of underlying social advantage or disadvantage, such as different positions in the social hierarchy."[245] Thus, while equity is not the same as equality, it is a commitment to increase the opportunity for health and human development for groups within society who have suffered discrimination.[246] This definition refers to the fairness with which resources (and thus health risks and outcomes) in a community are distributed. It is evident that the poor receive and use fewer resources than the rich in any community. Poor people face significant barriers to HIV/AIDS services in the forms of unaffordability, unavailability and low responsiveness of health services to their needs.

Equity in HIV/AIDS care requires that "hard to reach" groups have equal access to HIV/AIDS prevention, treatment (including drugs), care and support. These groups include people living in poverty (especially poor women), sex workers, IDUs, ethnic minorities, migrants, people living in remote rural areas, people of different sexual orientation, orphans and others who live on the margins of society. As discussed in Section 1, these groups are among the most vulnerable to HIV/AIDS.

As of 2005, only 16% of the people living with HIV in Asia in need of ART had access to such therapy.[247] Even with increased efforts to scale up the care and treatment of people living with HIV, not everyone in need can access ART immediately. Although progress has been made in reducing the costs of ARV therapy in the developing world, governments and the private sector need to step up efforts to ensure that treatment reaches those in greatest need. Initial assessments suggest that, despite efforts to scale up access to ART, these therapies are not reaching vulnerable and poor populations. In many countries, ART remains largely concentrated in urban areas, leaving rural populations underserved or forcing them to travel long distances. Stigma and discrimination can also limit the access of vulnerable populations, such as sex workers, IDUs and MSM, to ART or lead to services that are unresponsive to the needs of these populations.[248]

As the HIV/AIDS epidemic progresses, it is becoming clear that gender inequality is increasingly shaping the contours of the epidemic. As discussed above, biology and gender inequality intersect to make women especially vulnerable to infection with HIV. Differences in the prevalence of HIV among women as compared with men thus reflect gender norms and the underlying distribution of power in society rather than individual choice. The powerful influence of gender inequality is also witnessed in the concentration of HIV infection among men and women who do not conform to dominant gender roles, such as MSM and sex workers.

Differences in the burden of HIV/AIDS from gender inequality are thus recognized as being unfair and unjust. Inequalities in access by women as compared with men to appropriate testing, counselling and treatment services can affect the rate at which women progress from HIV infection to AIDS. Similarly, MSM remain largely underserved by efforts to expand efforts to HIV testing, counselling and treatment. This suggests that health systems, in general, and HIV/AIDS interventions, in particular, may be unable to successfully respond to women's biological and social vulnerability to HIV/AIDS, as well as that of other groups marginalized by prevailing gender norms. To date, indications of gender bias in the distribution of ART are few. However, the focus on expanding efforts to prevent mother-to-child transmission of HIV/AIDS can miss non-pregnant women and girls.[249] Efforts are therefore required—both from within and beyond the health sector—to address the differences in the burden of HIV and AIDS among men and women arising from gender inequality.

The specific problems related to infected and affected children must be addressed. Without adequate nutrition, education, emotional and financial support, these children—who are the future of a nation—will be less able to contribute to the future social and economic development of their nation. Governments, international donor agencies, NGOs, faith-based organizations (FBOs), and the private sector must work together to ensure gender-sensitive education, adequate nutrition, and emotional and financial support to these very needy children.

Human rights

Human rights refer to an internationally agreed upon set of principles and norms that are spelt out in treaties, declarations and recommendations at international and regional levels. As HIV/AIDS affects so many aspects of life, many issues related to human rights are pertinent to HIV/AIDS prevention and control. A number of rights and general principles relevant to protecting human rights in the context of HIV/AIDS are outlined in various international human rights treaties. Of particular concern is the right to health for men and women, boys and girls. The Universal Declaration of Human Rights spells out the right to the highest attainable standard of physical and mental health. The Convention on the Elimination of All Forms of Discrimination Against Women (CEDAW) articulates a woman's right to health, including the protection of women who are infected with and affected by HIV.[250] Countries that ratify CEDAW agree that they will "take all appropriate measures to eliminate discrimination against women in the field of health care" to ensure that women and men have equal access to health services. The United Nations Convention on the Rights of the Child (CRC) reaffirms the right of children to health. These commitments have been reaffirmed in numerous regional treaties. To date, every country in the world is party to at least one human rights treaty that addresses health-related rights.[251]

In recognition of the dynamic relationship between human rights and HIV/AIDS, the International Guidelines on HIV/AIDS and Human Rights were drafted in the late 1990s. These 12 guidelines translate international human rights principles into practical strategies for action. In 2002, the guidelines were revised to respond to emerging issues. In particular, Guideline 6 on "access to prevention, treatment, care and support" was revised to reflect growing access to ART. The guideline was revised to place universal access to HIV/AIDS prevention, treatment and care at the heart of efforts to respect, protect and fulfil human rights related to health. More recently, world leaders reaffirmed

---

Box 4: HIV, human rights and the Siracusa Principles

A rights-based approach to HIV prevention, treatment and care is sometimes pitted against a concern for public health. The concern for autonomy, privacy and consent, among others, which are embedded in human rights, has been described as being privileged over public health measures, such as the routine or widespread testing for HIV. A rights-based approach does not oppose such public health measures aimed at preventing and controlling HIV/AIDS. Rather, the focus is on guaranteeing basic rights such as consent, confidentiality, information and protection from HIV-related discrimination and stigma. This approach is seen to be central to efforts that aim to increase people's willingness to be tested and receive treatment for HIV/AIDS.

This debate sits alongside wider concerns for balancing human rights and public health. The international community has recognized the right of governments to limit human rights in the interest of public health. Yet even in these circumstances, governments must abide by the Siracusa Principles. Governments must ensure that: the restriction is provided for and carried out in accordance with the law; the restriction is in the interest of a legitimate objective of general interest; the restriction is strictly necessary in a democratic society to achieve the objective; less intrusive and restrictive means are not available to reach the same objective; and the restriction is not drafted or imposed arbitrarily.

Source: Jurgens, Cohen n.d.; World Health Organization 2002a.

that "the full realization of all human rights and fundamental freedoms for all is an essential element in the global response to the HIV/AIDS pandemic."

Available evidence indicates that translating these principles into national legislation and a rights-based approach in HIV prevention and control at the country level has been uneven. Efforts to monitor the International Guidelines on HIV/AIDS and Human Rights at the country level have identified major gaps in implementation.[252] A more punitive approach to HIV continues to characterize much HIV-related policy among countries in the Region. This approach may include the criminalization of actions that 'intentionally' transmit HIV and mass testing for HIV without consent, for example.[253] Research has demonstrated that these approaches tend to promote stigma and deter people from coming forward for testing and treatment for HIV. As such, they may reduce the effectiveness of HIV prevention and control. Box 4 discusses a rights-based approach to HIV prevention, treatment and care as compared with a concern for public health.

Non-discrimination is a key concept within human rights. It forbids "any discrimination in access to health care and the underlying determinants, as well as to means and entitlements for their procurement, on the grounds of race, colour, sex, language, religion, political or other opinion, national or social origin, property, birth, physical or mental disability, health status (including HIV/AIDS), sexual orientation, civil, political, social or other status, which has the intention or effect of nullifying or impairing the equal enjoyment or exercise of the right to health".[254] However, due to stigma and discrimination, PLWH and those affected by the epidemic are often unable to live lives of equality, dignity and freedom. For example, some employers require HIV testing as a condition of employment. This practice discriminates against workers based on their expected future decline in productivity or increase in health care costs. Such discrimination, based on a condition that is unrelated to the worker's present abilities, is inefficient because it deprives the country of possible contributions made to the economy. Indeed, stigma and discrimination are recognized as among the greatest barriers to preventing new infection and easing the impact of the epidemic. Stigma and discrimination often violate the rights of PLWH on the basis of their HIV status, including the right to privacy, confidentiality, access to acceptable health care, reproductive and sexual health, employment, education, freedom of movement and the right to travel.[255]

States are responsible for the progressive realization of human rights, including the right to health. The various state obligations with respect to HIV/AIDS have been detailed at the international level.[256] These obligations are guided by four broad principles relating to health care and the underlying determinants of health: availability, accessibility, acceptability and quality of care (Box 5). This framework intersects with the obligation of states to respect, protect and fulfil human rights, which includes regulating the actions of non-state actors to ensure the right to health is realized.[257] Fulfilment of a government's obligations with

---

Box 5: HIV/AIDS and the accountability of states

When evaluating the right to health in HIV prevention and control, four criteria may be used:

Availability: Well-functioning prevention, treatment, support and care services for HIV/AIDS are adequately available.

Accessibility: Prevention, treatment, support and care services for HIV/AIDS are accessible to all, encompassing four dimensions: non-discrimination, physical accessibility, economic accessibility (affordability) and information accessibility.

Acceptability: Prevention, treatment, support and care services for HIV/AIDS are respectful, culturally appropriate, gender-sensitive and honour the confidentiality of all patients.

Quality: Prevention, treatment, support and care services for HIV/AIDS are scientifically and medically appropriate and of good quality.

Source: World Health Organization. 2002a.

regard to a person's right to non-discrimination, health, information, education, employment, social welfare and public participation, among others, is crucial to reducing vulnerability to HIV infection and to ensuring humane care and support for those infected with and affected by HIV.[258]

A human rights agenda places the individual at the centre of any health policy, programme or legislation. This approach strongly figures in the increasing involvement of people living with HIV, people who are affected by the epidemic, and communities in general. The "greater involvement of people living with HIV/AIDS" (GIPA) approach recognizes the right of PLWH, youth and other vulnerable communities to participate actively and meaningfully in all aspects of programmatic and policy-related responses to the epidemic. The GIPA approach aims to create policies and programmes that are informed by the experiences of PLWH and other vulnerable communities rather than by the perceptions of policy-makers and bureaucrats. The participation of PLWH and other vulnerable groups can effectively challenge stigma and discrimination, thereby complementing other preventive measures. Participatory approaches can also play an important role in holding governments to account. A rights-based approach, one that addresses stigma and discrimination, removes legal obstacles and other barriers to prevention, treatment and care for HIV/AIDS and enables the meaningful involvement of PLWH and other vulnerable groups, can thus create an environment of trust and respect that is critical to tackling the epidemic.

4. How can health professionals address poverty and gender concerns in HIV/AIDS?

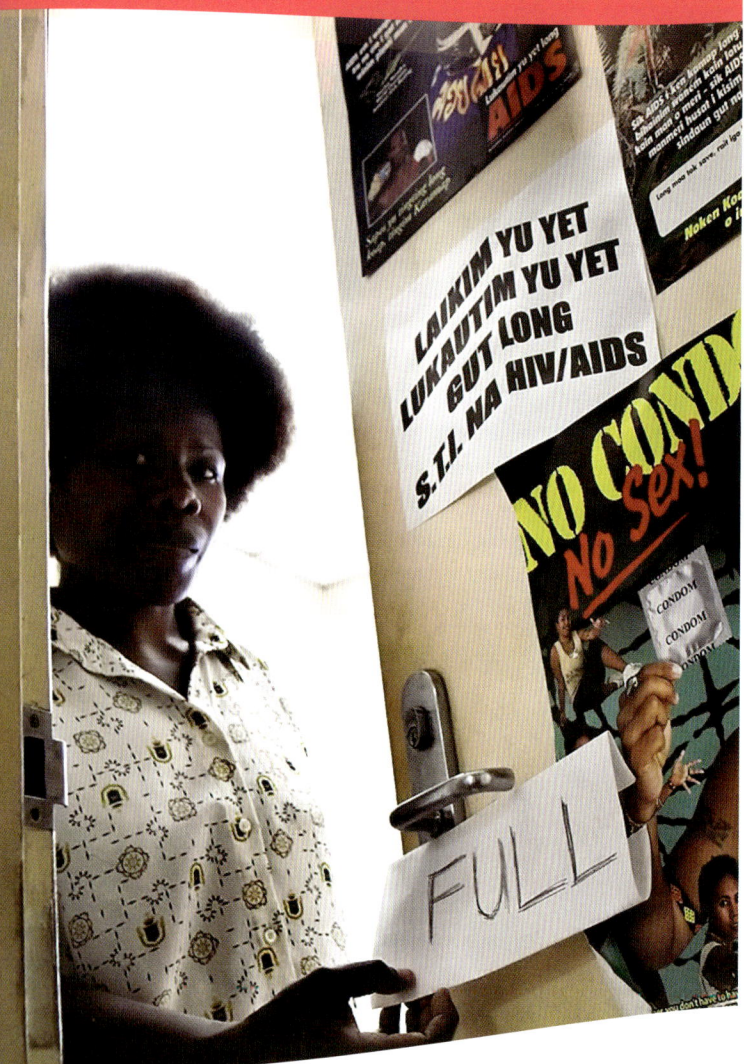

Integrating Poverty and Gender into Health Programmes: *A Sourcebook for Health Professionals*
Module on HIV/AIDS

4. How can health professionals address poverty and gender concerns in HIV/AIDS?

This section of the module examines how health professionals can address poverty and gender concerns in HIV/AIDS policies, programme planning and implementation, and service delivery.

Policy level

Establishing an enabling policy environment is crucial to the delivery of effective, equitable and gender-sensitive prevention, treatment and care of HIV/AIDS. The principles articulated in health policies and laws guide the formulation and implementation of HIV/AIDS-related plans and programmes. Reviewing the policy environment to ensure that health policies, including legislation, are based on the best available evidence and enable the realization of human rights for both men and women can help ensure that HIV prevention and control efforts address poverty- and gender-related concerns.

International policies

At the international level, many HIV/AIDS-related policies are grounded in a commitment to human rights. Besides the various international human rights treaties, numerous international initiatives set out the commitments, actions and goals agreed upon at the international level to stop and reverse the spread of HIV/AIDS. Halting and beginning to reverse the spread of HIV/AIDS, malaria and other diseases by 2015 is a target under Goal 6 of the eight Millennium Development Goals (MDGs). During the United Nations Special Session of the General Assembly on HIV/AIDS (UNGASS) in 2001, the international community pledged their unanimous support to the Declaration of Commitment on HIV/AIDS. The Declaration of Commitment articulates a number of priorities to address factors that make individuals particularly vulnerable to HIV infection, including underdevelopment, poverty, lack of empowerment of women, lack of information and/or the means for self protection, and all types of sexual exploitation of women, girls and boys, including that for commercial reasons.

The Declaration of Commitment articulated numerous goals in the following areas: leadership; prevention; care, support and treatment; HIV/AIDS and human rights; reducing vulnerability; children orphaned and made vulnerable by HIV/AIDS; alleviating the social and economic impact; research and development; HIV/AIDS in conflict and disaster-affected regions; resources; and, follow-up. The goals and targets of the UNGASS on HIV/AIDS serve as a benchmark for global action and blueprint for realizing the HIV-related MDGs.[259] Box 6 outlines MDG 6 and related targets and the UNGASS global targets for low- and middle-income countries.

The 2006 UN General Assembly High Level Meeting on HIV/AIDS, which followed up on the implementation of the Declaration of Commitment on HIV/AIDS, pledged global support for scaling up efforts and moving towards the goal of universal access to comprehensive HIV prevention, treatment, care and support by 2010. This commitment to universal access is considered integral to efforts to meet the MDGs and halt the spread of the HIV pandemic. This further reinforces a number of international commitments, including the Declaration of Commitment. Importantly, it builds on the commitment of the Group of Eight (G8) to "work with WHO, UNAIDS and other international bodies to develop and implement a package for HIV prevention, treatment and care, with the aim of coming as close as possible to universal access to treatment for all those who need it by 2010". The United Nations General Assembly subsequently endorsed this commitment in 2005.[260] Efforts towards the goal of universal access are guided by a number of basic principles: services should be equitable, accessible, affordable, comprehensive and sustainable.[261]

A number of international initiatives have recognized that unequal gender relations fuel the epidemics and particularly enhance the vulnerability of women and girls to HIV infection. Beyond their broad commitment to gender equality through international human rights instruments, the international community has committed itself to tackling gender inequality and enabling the empowerment of women as key strategies in the response to AIDS.

At the XIV International AIDS Conference in Barcelona in 2002, a Women's Bill of Rights was drafted. The first working draft of the Bill was developed and presented at the International AIDS Conference in Bangkok, Thailand, in 2004 (see Box 29 in Section 6, Tools). The International Community of Women (ICW) identified 12 ways to improve the situation of women living with HIV and AIDS throughout the world (see Box 28 in Section 6, Tools, resources and references).

At the global level, the Commission for Social Determinants of Health, which was set up by WHO, aims to draw attention to the impact of social determinants on producing and sustaining inequalities in health. The Commission's mandate includes recommending strategies to improve the health of poor men and women, boys and girls, by addressing the social determinants of health.[262]

HIV/AIDS has also been articulated as a poverty reduction priority in the Poverty Reduction Strategy Papers (PRSPs).[263] The PRSPs theoretically provide an example of a cross-sectoral approach to tackling social determinants of health. Thus, the process provides a mechanism for integrating HIV/AIDS into national development planning. A recent desk-based review of 22 PRSPs concluded that the extent to which HIV/AIDS was mainstreamed into PRSPs was mixed. In general, analysis of HIV/AIDS was weak and the links between poverty and HIV/AIDS were rarely examined in depth. The interaction between gender inequality and HIV/AIDS was noticeably absent from many PRSPs and few included sex-disaggregated data or gender-related goals and targets. The PRSPs of Asian countries included less coverage on HIV/AIDS than those of African countries. The PRSPs for Cambodia, the Lao People's Democratic Republic and Viet Nam include some analysis of HIV/AIDS.[264] The PRSP for Mongolia does not discuss HIV/AIDS in the main text, but targets for HIV/AIDS are included in the summary of the MDGs for Mongolia.[265] The interrelationship between poverty and HIV is further illustrated by

---

Box 6: Global blueprint to stop and reverse the spread of HIV: MDG 6 and the UNGASS global targets for low- and middle-income countries

MDG 6: Combat HIV/AIDS, malaria, and other diseases

Target 7: Have halted by 2015 and begun to reverse the spread of HIV/AIDS
- 18. HIV prevalence among pregnant women aged 15 to 24
- 19. Condom use rate of the contraceptive prevalence rate
- 19a. Condom use at last high-risk sex
- 19b. Percentage of 15- to 24-year-olds with comprehensive correct knowledge of HIV/AIDS
- 19c. Contraceptive prevalence rate
- 20. Ratio of school attendance of orphans to school attendance on non-orphans aged 10 to 14

Declaration of Commitment on HIV/AIDS: global targets, low- and middle-income countries, 2005
- Increase total annual expenditure to US$ 7 billion–US$ 10 billion.
- By 2005, at least 90% of young people aged 15 to 24 correctly identify ways of preventing HIV transmission. This figure should climb to 95% by 2010.
- By 2005, 80% of HIV-positive women receive antiretroviral prophylaxis.
- By 2005, 50% of people with advanced HIV infection receive antiretroviral therapy.
- Reduce by 25% the rate of HIV infection among young people aged 15 to 24 in the most affected countries by 2005 and globally by 2010.
- Reduce the proportion of infants who are infected by HIV-positive mothers by 20% by 2005 and 50% by 2010.

Source: World Bank, 2007; United Nations General Assembly 2006.

> **Box 7: AIDS and the Millennium Development Goals**
>
> HIV/AIDS epidemics are reducing the chances of achieving the Millennium Development Goals and targets for many heavily burdened countries.
>
> The epidemics undermine poverty reduction efforts by sapping economic growth, thus hampering efforts to reach **Goal 1, to eradicate extreme poverty and hunger**. Educational opportunities recede as HIV/AIDS redirects household income to medical care and funerals, thus affecting the chances of reaching **Goal 2, to achieve universal primary education**. In addition to killing millions of women, HIV/AIDS adds to the caregiving burdens of women and girls, reducing their chances of pursuing education and paid work, and hence undermining **Goal 3, to promote gender equity and empower women**. HIV-positive women face many forms of discrimination and psychological and physical abuse. In many countries with the highest adult HIV prevalence, AIDS has lead to a rise in infant and under-five mortality, thereby reducing many countries' chances of reaching **Goal 4, to reduce child mortality**. The disease also reduces the chances of reaching **Goal 5, to reduce maternal mortality**. Research has found that maternal mortality is higher among women with HIV than among those who are HIV negative. HIV infection also directly increases the risks of developing tuberculosis and adversely affects the chances of contending with malaria and other diseases, as part of **Goal 6, to combat HIV/AIDS, malaria and other diseases**. One target of **Goal 7, to ensure environmental stability**, offers an opportunity to improve the lives of at least 100 million slum dwellers by 2020. However, HIV/AIDS is likely to threaten many millions of them. All goals depend on **Goal 8, to develop a global partnership for development**. This goal links donors, governments, civil society and the private sector. HIV/AIDS is undermining progress here, for example, through its decimation of countries' skilled workforces. Providing access to essential medicines is a key target. Expanding HIV/AIDS treatment will be vital to progress.
>
> Source: World Health Organization 2004b.

how HIV threatens progress towards each of the MDGs (Box 7).

National policies

National-level political commitment to respond to the HIV/AIDS epidemic is essential for programme success. Such commitment needs to be translated into concrete national policies that ensure the realization of international goals and targets for HIV/AIDS within the framework of human rights and gender equality. Enacting and refining legislation, policies and plans across national governments can create a policy environment that is supportive of realizing poverty and gender concerns. This can, in turn, enable effective and equitable programmatic initiatives at the national and local levels.[266]

The centrality of national-level responses in the response to AIDS is illustrated in the "Three Ones" principles, endorsed at a high-level meeting in 2004. Led by the affected countries, the principles commit donor agencies and developing countries to work together more effectively on a country-by-country basis, to achieve the best use of resources and ensure rapid results. An HIV/AIDS action framework provides the basis for coordinating the work of all partners and promotes an enabling environment across multiple sectors.[267] The Three Ones are:

- one agreed HIV/AIDS action framework that provides the basis for coordinating the work of all partners;
- one national AIDS coordinating authority, with a broad-based multisectoral mandate; and
- one agreed country-level monitoring and evaluation system.

Countries with relatively high HIV prevalence have established central management units for HIV/AIDS care and treatment through the national AIDS programmes or national AIDS coordinating committees. These national bodies are working to develop a national standardized, unified and coherent approach to HIV/AIDS care and treatment that is in line with the Three Ones. Global experience shows that the following elements are most central to effective national HIV prevention programmes:[268]

- promoting general awareness-raising activities to provide information and counter negative reactions among the larger population;
- developing partnerships that are multisectoral and multilevel in order to deliver programmes and services across a range of contexts;
- promoting community ownership of programmes, and building upon the will of groups and individuals to contribute to national HIV prevention efforts;
- encouraging greater integration between prevention and care to reduce costs;
- developing programmes to reduce discrimination and stigmatization;
- promoting action to build societal resistance to HIV transmission; and
- providing programmes to reduce systematic vulnerability of particular individuals, groups and segments of society.

More recently, there has been a drive to translate the global commitment to universal access to HIV prevention, treatment care and support into national targets. The aim is to establish ambitious yet feasible 2010 targets that will galvanize political commitment and national ownership. As at the international level, the movement towards universal access is not new. Rather, it builds on past experience and aims to infuse existing initiatives with new momentum, including political and financial commitment. This approach is comprehensive, integrating HIV prevention, treatment and care, and is built on the pillars of the Three Ones.[269]

Within these broad strategies, efforts are required to translate general commitments to poverty and gender concerns into HIV/AIDS policies and programmes. For example, to integrate the principle of equity into efforts to achieve universal access, WHO and UNAIDS recommend the following: a broadly representative ethics advisory board should be established at the national level (in line with structures set up under the Three Ones principles); public dialogue with a wide variety of stakeholders should be carried out on equity of access to prevention, treatment and care for HIV/AIDS; and policies and corresponding evaluation systems should be developed to specifically promote equality.[270]

HIV-related goals and policies typically aim to prevent and treat HIV/AIDS within the population as a whole, with HIV-related targets and indicators often expressed as national or population averages. Research suggests that these national targets can be achieved in the aggregate without necessarily improving the health of poor and marginalized households and communities.[271] Goals and policies for HIV prevention, treatment and care should clearly articulate a concern for marginalized groups in order to effectively guide efforts to reduce the burden of HIV among the poor. Moreover, goals and policies should be formulated specifically to improve the health of men and women, boys and girls, in order to reduce inequalities in the burden of HIV/AIDS, AIDS-related mortality and access to prevention and treatment services for HIV/AIDS, as well as limit the impoverishing effects of AIDS-related illness and treatment-seeking among poor men and women. Clearly defined objectives can then be used to guide policy and project design, implementation and monitoring.[272]

Because HIV/AIDS affects all areas of life and is driven by determinants that lie beyond the health sector, a coordinated response to the epidemic must include economic, political and social efforts. The need for a cross-sectoral response to the HIV/AIDS epidemic is most clearly illustrated by the vulnerability of women and girls to HIV infection and the impact of HIV/AIDS on them. Their vulnerability to infection is rooted in both biological and socioeconomic factors. As such, legislation and policies need to be revised and enacted to address these complex elements. Women and girls should be ensured equal access to: information and education, economic resources and productive assets, protection from violence and political empowerment, among others.[273]

A broad cross-sectoral strategy to reduce inequalities in income, education attainment and nutritional status, among others, can enhance pro-poor HIV/AIDS prevention, treatment and care. Some countries have set up independent national human rights institutions (NHRIs) to promote and protect human rights. These institutions help to reduce discrimination and improve the quality of life of PLWH. They recognize HIV/AIDS not only as a health issue, but also as a human rights issue because of its serious civil, cultural, economic, political and social implications. Establishing partnerships with women's organizations and the active participation of men and women living with HIV/AIDS can also enable efforts to enact and implement gender-equality policies.

Financing

Numerous international initiatives to raise the level of funding for HIV prevention, treatment and care are currently underway. For example, the Global Fund to Fight AIDS, Tuberculosis and Malaria has increased funding for HIV-related programmes and projects. The Global Fund has provided funding for HIV/AIDS projects addressing prevention, surveillance and STI diagnostics in 11 countries in the Pacific. In Papua New Guinea, the Global Fund supports a comprehensive approach to HIV/AIDS treatment, care and support.[274] Funding has likewise been provided for national HIV/AIDS programmes in Cambodia, China, the Lao People's Democratic Republic, Mongolia, the Philippines and Viet Nam.[275]

At the country level, more efficient and equitable allocation of financial and human resources within the health sector can enhance the pro-poor impact of increased resources. Box 8 contains a checklist for mobilizing resources for HIV/AIDS programmes with emphasis on issues related to poverty and gender.

More equitable allocation of resources can be complemented by a number of additional principles regarding the financing of HIV/AIDS prevention, treatment, care and support. Many of these approaches seek to shift the financial burden of HIV/AIDS from PLWH and those affected by the epidemic, particularly those who are poor and marginalized, to society more broadly. Subsidizing prevention efforts that have proven to be effective in halting the spread of HIV, such as improving access to male and female condoms and needle exchange programmes, can support poor men and

---

Box 8: Mobilizing resources and providing opportunities for people infected with or affected by HIV/AIDS

- Identify the key stakeholders to work on HIV/AIDS programmes.
- Focus on vulnerable groups and those living on the margins of society who are infected with or affected by HIV/AIDS. Try to involve them in developing the HIV/AIDS programme.
- Involve others in the programme's development (particularly those living with HIV/AIDS).
- Assess the available financial resources and develop a financial plan for the programme.
- Ascertain the goods and services that will be required.
- Develop partnerships with the government, NGOs, donor and development agencies, the private sector, communities and people infected with or affected by HIV/AIDS.
- Develop a strategic planning process involving key stakeholders (e.g. government leadership, community participation, PLWH, and donor and development agencies); confirm existing resources; and mobilize additional resources (e.g. through mobilizing new partnerships, developing technical support networks, and raising funds through involving development agencies.

Adapted from Joint United Nations Programme on HIV/AIDS 2000b.

women in taking actions to protect themselves from HIV. Efforts to develop universal health insurance schemes or other risk-pooling measures can assist HIV-infected and -affected families with the cost of health care. Having poor people pay for their health care out of pocket only creates more poverty and ultimately affects the economic and social development of a nation. Box 9 describes a prepayment health insurance scheme for PLWH in Rwanda.

Equitable pricing for anti-HIV medications can likewise improve access to ART for poor individuals and households. For example, international efforts to conduct negotiations with pharmaceutical companies have led to significant decreases in the price of certain combinations of generic anti-HIV drugs for low- and middle-income countries. In addition, generic drug manufacturers (notably in Brazil, India and Thailand) are producing ARV drugs and offering them in their domestic markets and, in some cases, for export.[276] This example points to the pivotal role the private sector can play in the response to AIDS. Box 10 provides an example of an innovative strategy whereby a company financed the cost of ART for its employees and their spouses. Recognizing the importance of securing sustained access to ART for poor individuals who are unable to afford treatment, WHO promotes the provision of ARVs free of charge at the point of service delivery.[277]

Programme planning

Experience suggests that effective national responses are those designed to meet the specific needs of the particular country, address situations that make people vulnerable to HIV and its

---

Box 9: Prepayment scheme for health care for PLWH in Rwanda

In Rwanda, the prevalence of HIV in pregnant women is estimated to range from 13% in Kigali to less than 3% in some rural areas. A recent proposal to the Global Fund to Fight AIDS, Tuberculosis and Malaria identified lack of interaction between the population and the health system as a key obstacle to HIV/AIDS prevention and control in Rwanda. To improve the accessibility of health services in Rwanda, the proposal outlined a strategy to reduce the financial burden of seeking care and to enhance the quality and performance of health services.

In areas where out-of-pocket user fees are common, analysis has shown that average treatment costs may be as much as the median monthly income of a rural household in Rwanda. This can contribute to the low utilization of health services in rural areas, where households seek care for fewer than 60% of disease episodes. The proposal built on the successful experience with community-based health insurance in other areas of the country to address these issues.

Previous experience shows that households covered by the community-based health insurance scheme accessed health care services three to five times more than non-members. To extend coverage of community-based health insurance, the Global Fund financed the full cost of membership to the insurance scheme for very poor households, people living with HIV/AIDS, and members of vulnerable groups. It has also financed 50% of the membership costs for all rural households in the six provinces covered by the proposal. The community-based health insurance scheme enjoys strong backing from a number of donor agencies and is the subject of a draft national law that would extend health insurance coverage to all families, with particular emphasis on vulnerable groups. Coupled with efforts to improve the quality and performance of health services, this approach is expected to improve the accessibility of health services in Rwanda, thereby strengthening efforts to curb the HIV/AIDS epidemic.

Sources: Joint United Nations Programme on HIV/AIDS and World Health Organization 2006a; Physicians for Human Rights 2006.

> **Box 10: Engaging the private sector in the response to AIDS: financing prevention and treatment for employees of a diamond mine in Botswana**
>
> In 1999/2000, Debswana, a diamond mining company in Botswana, carried out an institutional audit to ascertain the epidemic's impact on the company and its operations. It discovered that retirement due to ill health and AIDS-related deaths had risen markedly. Company hospitals were also recording more admissions of workers with HIV/AIDS-related conditions. A concerted response was called for.
>
> The audit analysed risk-reduction strategies, estimated costs associated with benefits, developed systems to monitor productivity, and considered potential treatment options. The result was a landmark policy to cover 90% of the costs of ARV treatment for workers and their spouses, and to require suppliers of goods and services to the company to have AIDS programmes in place. In addition, prevention measures were prioritized.
>
> Source: Joint United Nations Programme on HIV/AIDS 2002a.

impact, and make use of the unique strengths of the country's people and institutions. Taking examples from neighbouring countries' experiences or from a comprehensive set of "best known practices" and adapting them to the country's particular situation, can save time and increase the chances of achieving success. UNAIDS has drafted a four-module guide that can be used by countries that want to develop an HIV/AIDS strategy.[278] Box 11 describes how the Swedish Agency for International Development Cooperation (Sida) extends support for the mainstreaming of HIV issues and actions into the health sector.

It is also becoming increasing clear that effective and equitable national-level responses to HIV/AIDS need to consider the different needs of men and women, boys and girls in designing plans and interventions.[279] Integrating gender concerns into HIV/AIDS programming requires gender analysis of sex-disaggregated data (see page 70) and the active participation of nongovernmental organizations, community groups committed to gender equality and men and women living with HIV/AIDS in all aspects of programme planning. Strengthening the responsiveness of the health system to respond to the needs of men and women, both as service providers and patients, is also needed.[280]

Gender concerns need to be integrated as a core element of programme planning and implementation. Approaches to gender in health programming can be characterized as falling along a continuum, ranging from gender-unequal, which harm the cause of gender equality, to gender-transformative or -empowering, which aim to address the socioeconomic factors that determine the vulnerability of men and women to infection.[281] This typology is elaborated in Box 12. It is useful to keep this typology in mind while reviewing the various examples described in the sections that follow.

Prevention, treatment and care services

This section discusses prevention, voluntary counselling and testing (VCT), antiretroviral therapy and home-based care.[282] Figure 11 illustrates the main domains and elements of HIV comprehensive care. This approach to HIV prevention, treatment, care and support forms the basis of efforts to scale up towards universal access.[283] Notably, universal access requires more than achieving 100% coverage of HIV-related services.[284] It needs renewed commitment to prevention in concert with scaled-up access to voluntary testing and counselling, treatment, care and support for those affected by AIDS. To cater to the diversity of HIV epidemics in different countries and communities, HIV strategies need to be tailored to local needs and conditions.

It is important to incorporate HIV/AIDS prevention and care into general health care services to the extent possible. This can help

> **Box 11: Planning for the health sector with HIV in mind: the case of Sida**
>
> The Swedish Agency for International Development Cooperation (Sida) has developed a useful strategic framework for its approach to HIV/AIDS and its effects on the health sector. The framework recognizes that women and men are affected differently and any response to HIV must address these differences. Programme officers must be aware of gender and equity dimensions when analysing the effects of HIV/AIDS on the health sector. In addition, poor people are particularly affected by HIV/AIDS, and ways to prevent and mitigate their risk need to be specifically addressed. The framework has four strategic goals.
>
> **Addressing immediate causes**
> 1. Prevention of HIV/AIDS
>   - sex education and services (to patient and others)
>   - control of sexually transmitted infections
>   - prevention of mother-to-child transmission
>   - improved blood routines
>   - harm reduction programmes
>
> **Addressing immediate effects**
> 2. Providing care, counselling and support
>   - creative response to increasing numbers of HIV/AIDS patients
>   - treatment of opportunistic infections
>   - provision of terminal care
>   - voluntary testing and counselling
>
> **Addressing underlying causes**
> 3. Enhancing political commitment
>   - monitoring the epidemic
>   - providing data to political leaders
>   - stimulating informed leadership
>
> **Addressing long term effects**
> 4. Protecting the health system
>   - promote planning to handle HIV/AIDS among health staff
>   - find ways to counteract burnout among staff
>   - overcome difficulties motivating people to work
>   - as medical doctors and nurses in severely HIV/AIDS-affected countries
>
> Source: Sodeco Social Development Consultants 2002.

ensure the access to services and reduce stigma attached with HIV prevention, treatment and care. However, specific and proactive efforts are required to ensure that HIV-related initiatives are pro-poor and gender sensitive. That is, HIV policies need to be translated into those that articulate a concern for poverty and gender into measurable outcomes. Box 23 (see Section 6, Tools) highlights some of the key strategies to ensure that the HIV/AIDS services are pro-poor and gender-sensitive.[285] Box 24 (see Section 6, Tools) comprises a tool to ensure that programmes and policies as well as their implementing agencies reflect gender sensitivity.

The following section presents information on innovative strategies that health professionals are employing to improve accessibility and equity in HIV prevention, treatment, care and support for poor men and women, boys and girls. These interventions are still in their early stages, and have not yet been evaluated rigorously or standardized.

However, they suggest some ways forward. This list of strategies is not exhaustive. The strategies need to be adapted and refined, based on further analysis and country-specific situations.

Gaining the support of partner organizations (such as donor, policy, or community-based non-profit organizations) can strengthen gender-responsive HIV/AIDS programmes. Teaming up with other organizations that endorse efforts to change gender biases is useful for three reasons: helps legitimize the work being done; provides staff with "allies" and resource persons; and provides the potential for increased funding. Such organizations may be mobilized through person-to-person communications, informational meetings or media campaigns.

Prevention

In an era of growing commitment for universal access to prevention, treatment, care and support

> **Box 12: Integrating gender concerns into HIV/AIDS programming**
>
> Approaches to gender equality in HIV/AIDS programming vary and have evolved over time with increasing understanding of the role that gender relations and norms play in HIV/AIDS epidemics. Recent analysis proposes that these approaches to gender concerns can be arranged along a continuum, ranging from those that 'harm' or reinforce negative gender stereotypes to those that empower women and girls. The following categories for gender-responsive HIV/AIDS programming have been proposed:
>
> **Harm (or gender-unequal):** These interventions are often based on stereotypical ideas of gender-related roles and responsibilities. For example, efforts to prevent mother-to-child-transmission have tended to focus on mothers, without considering the influence that male partners or husbands and mothers-in-law have on their ability to make choices. These approaches tend to reinforce the harmful effect of these stereotypes on the health of men and women. In many areas, efforts to extend treatment and care to people living with HIV/AIDS have become increasingly dependent upon unpaid home-based care, with different implications for women and men. The work associated with home-based care often falls disproportionately upon women and girls because of the gender norms that assign care-giving work to women.
>
> **Do no harm (or gender-neutral):** This approach seeks to eliminate assumptions and stereotypes that are damaging to men and women and restrict their ability to benefit from policy and programmatic responses to HIV/AIDS epidemics. Simply put, this approach aims to offer health services that are different when the needs of men and women differ, without treating them differently when their needs are the same. To this end, approaches are designed based on data of men and women's lives within a particular community or setting.
>
> **Gender-sensitive:** This approach recognizes that the different needs of men and women are based not only on their biological characteristics but also on their gendered roles, responsibilities and relationships. Gender-based roles, responsibilities and relationships also influence how men and women are able to respond to HIV-related programmes and initiatives. Thus, this approach acknowledges gender differences and designs services and interventions to meet the differential needs of men and women. However, it does not necessarily question why these differences arise or seek to change these relations to achieve more equality in status.
>
> **Empowering (or gender-transformative):** This approach aims to create more equitable relationships between men and women by challenging the underlying determinants of the gender-related differences between men and women. The need to effectively reach both men and women with HIV programming is recognized. This approach may include challenging dominant notions of masculinity and working with youth to shift gender relations. The approach seeks to enable equitable power dynamics between men and women to reduce their vulnerability to HIV/AIDS. Locating HIV/AIDS within the large socioeconomic context, this approach addresses the sources of men and women's unequal power, including their access to education and information, their access to and control over economic resources and assets, gender-based violence and political participation of men and women.
>
> Source: World Health Organization 2003e.

of HIV/AIDS, efforts to prevent HIV transmission need to be intensified. At present, prevention programmes reach an estimated 1% of MSM, 5.4% of IDUs and less than 20% of female sex workers in the Region.[286] Enhancing the coverage and scope of prevention efforts and introducing innovative programmes tailored to meet the needs of hard-to-reach populations can effectively reducing the rising rates of infection. The sections below explore these issues with a focus on poverty and gender concerns.

Defining populations at risk

When they develop HIV/AIDS prevention programmes, planners need to pay attention to local conditions and the particular epidemiological trends of HIV in the given country or region. As discussed above, people's vulnerability to HIV/AIDS need to be considered, particularly as it relates to issues of gender and poverty. Vulnerable population groups need to be identified and these groups and their issues incorporated when developing, implementing or evaluating HIV/AIDS programmes, agencies or services. Box 13 provides suggested steps for developing effective HIV/AIDS prevention programmes that pay attention to poverty and gender concerns. In addition, Box 27 (see Section 6, Tools, resources and references) provides a checklist of what a HIV/AIDS prevention programme should achieve.

Strategies for HIV/AIDS prevention

Young people

One approach to reaching young people with information about HIV/AIDS is to incorporate such programmes into schools and thus potentially reach large numbers of young people before they become sexually active. In addition, school policies and programmes can help many adults, including school personnel, parents, and the wider community, to cope with HIV. HIV prevention programmes can promote tolerance and respect for people infected with HIV, can reduce stigmatization of teachers and students affected by the virus and can offer them social support.

Ideally, school-based HIV prevention programmes should begin early, be phased by age group and sustained from early childhood through adolescence. This approach is particularly desirable in settings where attendance rates drop dramatically after primary school. Age-appropriate information should be integrated into life-skills education programmes at an early age, before children become sexually active.

Targeting schools located in poor areas and extending this approach to cover children who

Figure 11: Comprehensive HIV/AIDS care and support

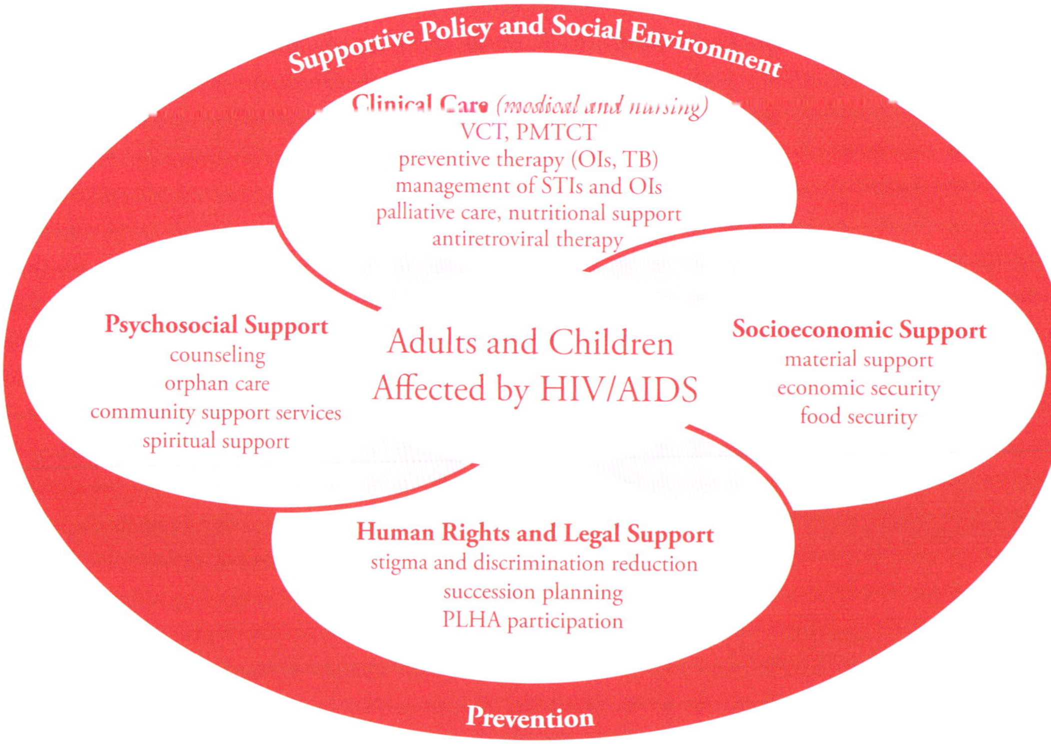

Supportive Policy and Social Environment

Clinical Care *(medical and nursing)*
VCT, PMTCT
preventive therapy (OIs, TB)
management of STIs and OIs
palliative care, nutritional support
antiretroviral therapy

Psychosocial Support
counseling
orphan care
community support services
spiritual support

Adults and Children Affected by HIV/AIDS

Socioeconomic Support
material support
economic security
food security

Human Rights and Legal Support
stigma and discrimination reduction
succession planning
PLHA participation

Prevention

Source: Family Health International 2004.

Box 13: Developing effective HIV/AIDS prevention programmes

Step 1. Collect evidence
- What are epidemiological trends in the area?
- What are the predominant routes of HIV transmission and risk behaviours that contribute to transmission?
- Who are the people most at risk for HIV infection?
- What are the particular needs of women and girls? Of children and infants, including with respect to possible mother to child transmission? Of men and boys?
- What is the share of people living in poverty who are infected with or affected by HIV?
- Do policies support or discriminate against people, especially those most at risk?

Step 2. Plan a prevention programme
Base your planning on the evidence collected in Step 1. You may likely not plan for all the initiatives identified in Step 2. However, the following are some common strategies for planning HIV prevention programmes:
- Involve key stakeholders, including people infected with and affected by HIV/IDS, NGOs, women and women's groups, government representatives, community leaders, religious leaders and others involved in HIV prevention and care.
- Make sure that vulnerable groups are involved in programme planning.
- Develop or adopt guidelines for purchasing, storing and distributing male and female condoms.
- Develop or adopt guidelines for safe collection, screening and transfusion of blood and organ transplantation.
- Develop or adopt guidelines for voluntary testing and counselling of HIV.
- Plan harm reduction programmes for injecting drug users.
- Plan programmes to discourage skin piercing practices and/or provide sterile skin piercing equipment.
- Plan programmes to eliminate female genital mutilation.

Step 3. Implement a prevention programme
Implementation should be based on data collected (Step 1) and the planning process (Step 2). That is, the HIV prevention programme should be implemented on sound evidence and good planning. The following are some important implementation issues:
- Involve vulnerable groups (see Steps 1 and 2) in implementing the programme.
- Ensure acceptability and geographical and financial accessibility for "hard to reach" groups.
- Ensure the HIV prevention programme meets the needs of the target population and provides services at times when people can access them.
- Ensure information, education and communication (IEC) materials are suited to the educational level of the target populations and produced in the local language.

Step 4. Monitor and evaluate
The following questions should be addressed to ensure effective monitoring and evaluation:
- Does the monitoring and evaluation plan enable disaggregation of the data and information by various relevant indicators of social exclusion, such as income, sex, location, ethnicity?
- Have you reached the target population? Has the programme contributed to safer HIV/AIDS prevention practices among those most in need?
- Have the prevention strategies used been effective (e.g. VCT programmes, IEC materials, theatre, condom promotion, safe injecting programmes)?
- What do staff think of the service? What works well, and what could be improved?
- What do users think of the service? What do they like best, and what would they like to see done differently?
- When will formal evaluation of the HIV prevention programme take place? Who will be the evaluator?

are unable to attend school, such as working children, will better ensure that poor children benefit from such approaches. In some settings, tailored approaches may be necessary to reach girls who are less likely to attend school or who have to leave school earlier than boys. Disseminating HIV prevention messages through non-formal education opportunities and channels, such as radio and peer educators, or at community centres, can ensure that these messages reach youth who are not in school. Involving working youth, those who live on the streets and other vulnerable groups among youth can ensure that prevention messages and strategies reflect their experiences and realities.

Prevention messages that urge abstinence, fidelity, consistent condom use, needle exchange programmes (for IDUs) and encourage and enable people to obtain prompt treatment for STIs have all helped prevent HIV infection. Evidence from several projects suggests that if young people have access to accurate information and the opportunity to discuss sexual health issues, they can and will change their behaviour to reduce the risk of HIV infection. For example, a school-based prevention project in China has established a network of teachers trained in life-skills and HIV/AIDS education. As a result, HIV/AIDS awareness has increased among local education officials, students, parents and the media.[287] Box 14 describes an innovative approach to reducing the vulnerability of marginalized boys and young men in India.

Gender-sensitive sexuality education (in and out of school) and youth-friendly services are characterized by:[288]

- educational and outreach efforts focused on motivating behavioural change, including responding to myths, expectations, gender-based double standards, and sociocultural factors;
- provision of information and services that are enabling, skill-building and problem-solving in orientation;

Box 14: Promoting sexual health and citizenship through participatory methods to reduce the vulnerability of marginalized boys and young men in West Bengal, India

Kishalaya is one of the biggest residential homes for children and youth in West Bengal. Police often bring children found living on the streets or at local railway stations to the home. Many of them are orphans who were abandoned by their families or who fled their homes to escape physical, sexual or emotional abuse. During their time on the streets or railway platforms, many were further abused, often arriving at Kishalaya in poor physical, mental and emotional health.

The boys and young men receive an education during their time at Kishalaya (many stay until 16 years of age). Praajak, a community organization, works with them on becoming responsible and productive citizens. Praajak's work is based on the view that, to overcome their past experiences, the boys and young men must develop new, positive views of themselves and others, including about what it means to be male. One way to do so is to learn how to establish trustful relationships with one another.

Praajak recognized that issues of sexual abuse had to be addressed; however, because of reservations among government staff overseeing Kishalaya, Praajak had to find an indirect way of tacking these issues. Every year, residents of Kishalaya put on performances for staff and members of the local community. The performances usually coincide with local festivals or mark various seasons of the year. Praajak staff used the stories and characters of these performances to encourage the boys and young men to discuss a broad range of issues. Participatory methods enable the boys and young men to speak the 'unspeakable', including some of their most difficult past experiences. Over time, the boys and young men become comfortable and willing to discuss emotional and sexual issues. Trustful relationships ensure that confidentiality is maintained.

Source: Wood *et al*. 2006.

- promotion of community-based mobilization for creating a supportive environment (Youth peer educators of both sexes can serve as community role models of gender equality and responsible behaviour.);
- wide availability of male and female condoms for sexually active youth in places where they can easily and anonymously access them;
- training of peer educators, health service providers and other outreach workers with an emphasis on gender-sensitive interpersonal communication and counselling skills for young people;
- provision of services that safeguard the rights to non-discrimination, confidentiality and privacy, particularly those that address the specific challenges men and women and boys and girls may face in negotiating voluntary, safer sexual relations or delaying sexual initiation; and
- raising of awareness on the implications of gender-based violence.

Gender-sensitive prevention messages need to be complemented by prevention methods that men as well as women can use. While condoms can effectively prevent the transmission of HIV through sexual intercourse, in many settings, women find it difficult to negotiate condom use with their male partners. Box 15 describes research initiatives that are seeking to respond to this situation by developing women-controlled alternatives.

Some research has concluded that promoting gender equity may be more effective during adolescence than in adulthood. Evidence suggests that young men frequently are more willing than adult men to consider alternative views about their roles in reproductive health and are in the process of forming their values—values that often shape lifelong patterns.[289] Male socialization has direct consequences for young men's health, including their risk-taking behaviours such as substance use, violence, and unsafe sexual practices. An analysis of boys with a gender equity perspective found that they were influenced by interactions with a relative, family friend or someone in their social circle who either modelled or supported non-traditional gender stereotypes.

Recognizing that both young men and women need comprehensive information on sexual and reproductive health, AIDS prevention programmes must target young men as well as young women.[290] Many young men know very little about the disease or about where to go for information. Gender-based norms may act as constraints, obliging them to impress their peers, hide their emotions, and show strength rather than weakness. However, evidence shows that young men, because of their age, can learn responsible sexual behaviour. Lessons from experience include the following:[291]

- Including young men in the response to HIV/AIDS can help contain the pandemic among young adults.
- Most young men practise responsible sexual behaviour and are willing to become involved in the response to AIDS.
- To enable young men to become partners in HIV/AIDS programmes, organizations need to reach out, creating opportunities and meeting young men's needs.

Sex workers

When used correctly and consistently, condoms can effectively prevent the spread of HIV

Box 15: Microbicides

Many women are prevented from negotiating condom use with their male partner. For them, prevention options that they can initiate are urgently needed. Research is being carried out to develop a microbicide—a cream, gel or film that would substantially reduce the transmission of HIV when applied topically to the vagina. Research into vaginal microbicides has been slow, but it is substantially widening the choice of protective interventions. If proven viable, these products would offer a powerful new prevention tool in the response to AIDS.

Source: *Microbicides*. Geneva, Joint United Nations Programme on HIV/AIDS, 2007.

and other STIs and protect against unwanted pregnancy. Promoting condom use is therefore an essential component of HIV/AIDS prevention programmes. Efforts to promote condom use among sex workers have been hampered by the fact that clients who do not wish to use condoms can often purchase sex from those who do not insist on condom use. As such, female sex workers who demand that their male clients use condoms may lose significant income, which could encourage them to forego condom use. Concurrently, the power dynamics between women sex workers and their men clients makes it difficult for sex workers to insist that their clients use condoms. The 100% condom use programme (100% CUP) is designed to overcome the challenges of promoting condom use among sex workers.

The goal of the 100% CUP is to reduce the transmission of HIV and STIs by ensuring that condoms are used:
- 100% of the time
- in 100% of risky sexual relations[292]
- in 100% of sex entertainment establishments in a large geographical area.

The 100% CUP is most effective in areas where HIV transmission is associated with sex work in sex entertainment establishments. In these places, commercial sex is negotiated and, at times, carried-out, under the general supervision of an owner and/or manager. The 100% CUP is planned and implemented in coordination with local authorities, including the police and public health office, the owners and managers of sex entertainment establishments, sex workers and NGOs, among other stakeholders. This multisectoral collaboration enables broad political support for the programme.

The aim of the 100% CUP is to create an environment that enables the consistent use of condoms in commercial sex. First, when the 100% CUP is implemented in a town, province or country, a woman sex worker can demand that her client use a condom, knowing that she will not lose the client to another sex worker in another establishment. That is, since all sex entertainment establishments in the given area require condom use, the client has no incentive to seek commercial sex elsewhere (no condom means no sex). Second, the 100% CUP employs a number of strategies to enable sex workers to negotiate condom use with their customers. Sex workers are educated on the benefits of condom use, methods to better negotiate condom use with clients, including ways of making condoms more sexually stimulating, and alternatives to unprotected sex. Most importantly, the 100% CUP places responsibility for ensuring consistent condom use with the owners and managers of the sex entertainment establishments. As a result, the owners and managers encourage and support sex workers to require condom use. In addition, the programme ensures a consistent supply of quality condoms to sex workers and their clients.

Consistent condom use is further supported through efforts to monitor the compliance of sex entertainment establishments. Owners and managers who do not comply with the programme are sanctioned, which can include warnings and temporary or permanent closure. STI services, including information, are offered to sex workers and their clients by the local public health facilities.[293]

Evidence to date confirms the effectiveness of this approach. In Cambodia, the 100% CUP has led to a doubling of condom use by brothel-base sex workers since 1998 and is attributed with halving the prevalence of HIV.[294] The use of condoms among establishment-based sex workers in pilot areas of China increased between 50.7% in Huangpi and 535.9% in Danzhou.[295] From 1996 to 1999, consistent condom use among the police in Cambodia was estimated to have increased from 65% to 85%.[296] About 66% of police and military in the Lao People's Democratic Republic stated that they always used condoms with commercial partners.[297] In many countries, the police are a key partner in HIV/AIDS prevention strategies, such as the 100% CUP.

Recent assessments of the 100% CUP in Cambodia may point to the need for strategies to ensure that the 100% CUP is responsive to the constraints that poverty and gender may place on sex workers. For example, in some areas, condoms are available free of charge to sex workers; in other areas, condoms must be purchased from health facilities, brothel owners or NGOs. When the financial cost of purchasing condoms rests on sex workers, they may be deterred from using them consistently. In addition, the low quality of care in some public STI clinics can deter female sex workers from seeking care.[298] Furthermore, the use of 'mystery clients' to monitor the condom use has drawn much criticism. A mystery client is a male volunteer who pretends to be a client and attempts to purchase sex without using a condom. Finally, it is important to remember that the 100% CUP is designed to improve condom use among female sex workers who work through sex entertainment establishments. To date, the programme has not been tailored to address the needs of male or transgendered sex workers or freelance female sex workers.[299]

Men who have sex with men

Sex between men occurs in all countries and societies. However, the extent to which sex between men is acknowledged varies among countries and communities, as does the level of stigma, discrimination and even criminalization of sex between men. With regards to HIV prevention, sex between men is of particular concern because it can involve anal sex, which when unprotected carries a high risk of HIV infection.[300] Men who have sex with men comprise men of diverse backgrounds, socioeconomic statuses, sexual orientations and gender identities. MSM do not necessarily identify themselves as homosexual and, indeed, in some countries are largely married or engage in heterosexual sex. This means that they may be instrumental in heterosexual transmission, too. In other countries, MSM may not be associated with a particular group or social identity. MSM, therefore, might not be a distinct group but rather a key part of the general population.[301]

In general, evidence is lacking on the diversity of experiences, gender identities and needs of MSM in relation to HIV prevention. Estimates suggest that at least 5%–10% of HIV infections globally occur in MSM. The prevalence of HIV in MSM has been estimated to range from less than 2% in some areas to over 20% in others.[302] However, experience shows that insufficient political will, stigma, discrimination and denial are key barriers to enhancing access to prevention services for MSM. Stigma and discrimination may deter men from revealing their sexual orientation or from seeking services for HIV prevention. A recent study reported that same sex remained criminalized in roughly 70 countries.[303] Conversely, government officials and the police may harass those offering HIV-related services to MSM. Globally, only about 10% of MSM have access to HIV prevention, treatment and care.[304] Because of this, efforts to improve access to HIV prevention for MSM need to create an environment that protects the rights of MSM in both law and practice and enables them to access prevention services tailored to meet their needs. When matched with sufficient scaling up of HIV prevention efforts, this approach has proven to be effective in preventing HIV infection among MSM. In addition, efforts are required to ensure that particularly vulnerable MSM, such as sex workers, have access to appropriate HIV prevention services. Here, civil society can play an important role, including the delivery of HIV prevention programmes and challenging discrimination and stigma.

Community-based prevention

Attention is increasingly turning to the role communities can play in halting the spread of HIV/AIDS. Community-based programmes for changing sexual behaviour have been shown to be effective in the prevention of HIV/AIDS and STI.[305] Such programmes are based on the mobilization and participation of community members in decisions that affect their health. This approach also aims to promote partnerships across a wide range of stakeholders, including community members, community-based organizations, health service providers and policy-makers, with a view to using community and health service resources and enhancing coordination and collaboration. While community-based initiatives may be effective in extending the reach of HIV/AIDS-related services, they do not, however, automatically benefit poor community members.

Communities tend to have multiple social hierarchies, with varying and unequal degrees of power and the potential for conflicts of interest. The differing interests within communities require recognition to ensure that better-off community members do not capture the benefits of community-based initiatives. Similarly, concerted effort is required to ensure that the women's interests are articulated in the planning and implementation of community-based interventions. Dividing men and women into separate groups may enable women to participate more freely than they would as part of a mixed-sex group. Box 16 describes the experience of a community-based AIDS education and prevention project in Uganda. Box 17 discusses how a community of vulnerable individuals—sex workers in India—created an environment that enabled them to protect themselves from HIV/AIDS through individual and group empowerment. Box 18 describes experience with Stepping Stones, a participatory training approach to behavioural change that is based on a shift in norms, particularly those related to gender inequality, at the community level.

Poverty- and gender-sensitive approaches to the prevention of mother-to-child transmission

WHO advocates a comprehensive strategy to prevent HIV infection in infants and young children. This strategy consists of: primary prevention of HIV among parents-to-be; prevention of unintended pregnancies among HIV-infected women; prevention of transmission of HIV from infected women to their infants; and care, treatment and support for mothers living with HIV, their children and families. This strategy is built on comprehensive maternal and child health (MCH) services, voluntary and confidential counselling and testing, ARV prophylaxis for the prevention of mother-to-child transmission (PMTCT), counselling and support for safe infant feeding, and optimal obstetrical practices. The strategy is underpinned by ensuring the provision of ART and care and support for women living with HIV, their children and families.[306] Integrating this strategy into reproductive health services can ensure a more holistic approach to the health of women and their children, including adequate prevention services for women who test negative for HIV.

Research has found that the risk of mother-to-child transmission (MTCT) can be reduced to 2%–4% by employing a combination of

---

Box 16: Family AIDS education and prevention in Uganda

The Islamic Medical Association of Uganda (IMAU) launched the Family AIDS Education and Prevention through Imams Project in 1992. The rationale behind the project was that prevention efforts would better succeed if the prevention messages were transmitted by trusted community members, such as religious leaders (Imams). The Imams asked community volunteers to train as their assistants. Their teams included one male and one female assistant and five female and male family HIV/AIDS workers. By 1997, IMAU had worked with leaders at 850 mosques and trained 6800 volunteers who had visited 102 000 homes. Evaluation showed significant increases in community members' correct knowledge concerning HIV/AIDS, including perinatal transmission and risks associated with unsterile circumcision. Condom use also increased, and people reported significantly lower numbers of sexual partners. The women family HIV/AIDS workers found that women were willing to confide in them about HIV/AIDS-related matters that they would not discuss with their husbands or the Imams. In addition, they played a critical role in reaching and educating teenage girls in the community.

Source: Alford *et al.* 2005.

> **Box 17: Women's health and HIV: a sex workers' project in Calcutta**
>
> The rate of HIV/AIDS infection in India is increasing rapidly. Most Indian women find it difficult to be assertive and negotiate safer sex. However, some sex workers are successfully negotiating safer sex as well as better treatment from society, including the police. In 1992, the STI/HIV Intervention Project (SHIP) in Calcutta set up a STI clinic to promote disease control and condom distribution among sex workers. However, the focus soon broadened to address issues of gender, class and sexuality. The sex workers themselves decide the programme's strategies.
>
> The project adopted the following strategies:
> - Peer educators wore uniforms and identification cards for greater social recognition. Training was organized to promote self-reliance and confidence among sex workers and to build respect for them in the community, replacing their image as 'fallen' women.
> - Peer educators made house visits to teach residents how to prevent STIs and HIV, how to access medical care, and how to question power structures that promote violence.
> - A survey conducted among long-term regular clients showed that only 52% had heard of HIV/AIDS and 73% had never used a condom. Alliances were formed between sex workers and clients to promote safer sexual practices.
> - In 1995, the sex workers formed a union to promote and enforce their rights. A code of conduct was developed and agreed to by the government.
>
> The outcomes and lessons from the project include the following:
> - SHIP has responded to needs as they arise. For example, sex workers have set up a credit and savings programme for self-employment.
> - Sex workers have set up a theatre group for communicating methods of negotiating safer sex with clients, the police and brothel owners in a non-threatening environment.
> - SHIP has worked with groups of (mainly) men, including brothel owners, clients and the police, to enlist their support for improved rights for sex workers.
> - The project has changed not only behaviour but also attitudes, such as how society views sexuality, social acceptance of sex work and legal ambiguities relating to it.
> - Sex workers have realized that their struggle is not very different from those of poor women in the informal sector. The struggle is against patriarchy and domination.
>
> Source: Nath, Madhubala. 2000. In: Tallis 2002.

interventions that include ARV prophylaxis given to women during pregnancy, labour and delivery and to the infant during the first week of life, obstetrical interventions including elective caesarean delivery prior to the onset of labour, and complete avoidance of breastfeeding. The fact that infection in infants and children in developed countries are increasingly rare points to the success of these interventions.[307]

However, the implementation of these interventions is constrained in many low- and middle-income countries, where elective caesarean delivery is rarely possible and it is often neither acceptable nor safe for a woman to not breastfeed. In these contexts, recent initiatives have focused on adopting effective ARV regimes beginning in the third trimester of pregnancy. This approach reduces the risk of transmission from 20%–45% among infected women who breastfeed (and from 15%–30% among those who do not breastfeed) to 2%–4%. However, a substantial risk of transmission remains during breastfeeding. Research on methods for reducing the transmission of HIV during breastfeeding continues.[308]

Experience has shown that PMTCT services need to focus on the needs of both men and women. Until recently, mothers alone had been the focus

> **Box 18: Exploring sex and sexual relationships to support behavioural change among individuals and communities: the experience of Stepping Stones**
>
> Stepping Stones is a participatory training methodology that has been used by numerous agencies in a variety of settings over the past 10 years. Stepping Stones was designed to address HIV/AIDS epidemics in sub-Saharan Africa by augmenting existing prevention methods and enhancing care at the community level for people living with HIV/AIDS. During the mid-1990s, mainstream prevention messages tended to focus on the dangers of HIV/AIDS and the benefits of ABC (abstinence, be faithful, and use a condom). These prevention messages were often directed towards women, with little consideration for local gender relations that may restrict the ability of women to take action to protect themselves from HIV/AIDS. In response, Stepping Stones was formulated to enable open discussions of the realities of sex and sexually relationships with communities, with particular attention to gender inequalities that frame these relationships. The aim was to equip individuals and communities with the communication and relationship skills to enable them to find their own solutions to both avoiding and coping with the threat of HIV/AIDS.
>
> To support and enable behaviour change, Stepping Stones is carried out over a number of sessions. Community members are separated by sex and age into groups to encourage open and frank discussion. Work with peer groups is complemented by periodic community meetings to share issues and create a space where 'special requests' can be made. These 'special requests' consist of asking others within the community to change attitudes and behaviours on specific, locally identified issues. This approach seeks to support and sustain individual behavioural change with shifts in community values and norms. Because challenging gender inequality is central to Stepping Stones, the involvement of women and men is actively supported.
>
> Recently, Action Aid commissioned a review of available monitoring and evaluation reports to assess the impact and effectiveness of Stepping Stones. The review found that there is "almost universal support for and appreciation of Stepping Stones as a behavioural change process". Almost all documents reviewed identified improvements in communication between spouses and between children and parents arising from Stepping Stone training. This outcome has been identified as particularly crucial in the context of HIV/AIDS, since discussing sex and sexual relationships are often difficult, yet pivotal, to efforts to prevent HIV/AIDS. Reviews of the Stepping Stones experience have also demonstrated a positive increase in knowledge of HIV, its causes and prevention.
>
> Stepping Stones has been credited with changes in knowledge and attitudes towards sexual behaviour, gender relations and people affected by HIV/AIDS. Evidence also suggests strong positive changes in behaviour, including increased uptake of condoms, reduced domestic violence, respect for women who refuse sex in marriage, improved communication between couples and parents and children, and more cooperation between them on household chores. While these results are promising and point to behaviour change that may limit the spread of HIV/AIDS, the review observes that they are also often generalized and based on self-reporting and/or observations following training initiatives. Therefore, there is a need for further monitoring and evaluation efforts.
>
> Source: ActionAid 2006.

of PMTCT services. However, men also play an important role in promoting and supporting effective PMTCT. To better reflect the joint responsibility of mothers and fathers in this chain of transmission, some organizations have replaced the term 'mother-to-child transmission' with the more gender-sensitive term 'parent-to-child transmission'.[309] Box 24 (see Section 6, Tools) contains a checklist to ensure gender-sensitive PMTCT.

In many parts of the world, voluntary testing and counselling are available in antenatal settings. Women are encouraged to learn their HIV status because of the risk of MTCT. However, if their status is divulged, many HIV-infected women face stigma, discrimination and possible violence, abandonment, neglect, destitution and ostracism.[310] Thus, HIV-infected women may be reluctant or unable to take advantage of interventions offered to protect their children from infection.[311] Many interventions, particularly the administration of ARV therapies, may make it difficult for HIV-positive women to keep their infection status a secret.

Partner notification and shared confidentiality of HIV status have become major public health strategies to reduce MTCT. Some studies have shown that providing HIV counselling and testing to both partners together can lead to greater acceptance and less abuse and abandonment of HIV-infected women. Problems may arise, however, when the HIV-infected woman fears domestic violence, and when the partner to be notified is the man she fears.[312] These problems suggest that there may be need to re-examine current public health requirements of disclosure and partner notification.[313] Involving the fathers and couple counselling, or shared confidentiality, could slow the rate of MTCT.[314]

Pro-poor and gender-sensitive voluntary HIV counselling and testing

HIV testing and counselling is recognized as a priority in national HIV programmes because it forms the gateway to HIV/AIDS prevention, care, treatment and support.[315] Experience shows that, with proper counselling, most people who know their HIV-positive status take measures to protect themselves and others.[316] However, people who do not know their HIV status are unable to receive appropriate health care services or access ART. An estimated 0.2% of adults in low- and middle-income countries had access to voluntary HIV counselling and testing (VCT) in 2003. At present, only 12% of people who want to be tested have the necessary access to do so.[317] Even when VCT services are available, many people are prevented from learning their HIV status because of stigma and discrimination. Estimates from countries with a high burden of HIV/AIDS suggest that less than 10% of people living with HIV know their status.

Further, in many developing countries, people are diagnosed and treated too late to enjoy the full benefits of ART.[318] Expanding the coverage of VCT and initiating a more diverse range of approaches is thus a key component of achieving universal access to prevention, treatment and care for HIV/AIDS.

The primary model of VCT in low- and middle-income countries has traditionally been based on initiation by the client. Depending on the context and level of HIV prevalence, client-initiated testing and counselling can be complemented with enhanced diagnostic HIV testing, provider-initiated testing and counselling and improved coverage of and better tools for testing HIV in infants and children.[319] The aim of provider-initiated testing and counselling is to enable people to be diagnosed and treated early enough to benefit from ART. HIV testing can be routinely offered in antenatal clinics, STI treatment centres, primary health care (PHC) facilities, hospitals, home-based care and community care services. Box 25 (see Section 6, Tools) provides an overview of the important activities related to poverty- and gender-sensitive VCT services. Further research indicates that young people would like access to HIV testing and counselling services if the services are confidential and inexpensive and if the results are reported honestly.[320]

As with client-initiated counselling and testing, provider-initiated counselling and testing must be guided by human rights and adhere to ethical principles. The three Cs, which have been advocated since HIV testing was launched in 1985, remain central to provider-initiated counselling and testing.[321] The three Cs are:
- ensure **c**onfidentiality
- be accompanied by **c**ounselling
- be conducted only with **c**onsent that is both informed and voluntary.

A policy environment that improves protection from stigma and discrimination and assures access to HIV prevention, treatment and care is a cornerstone of efforts to scale up access to HIV testing and counselling.[322] Box 19 describes recommendations by stakeholders on promoting more ethical and effective VCT in Asia.

Voluntary HIV counselling and testing is part of a holistic approach to promoting the sexual health of individuals, couples and communities at large. Voluntary counselling and testing programmes have increased the adoption of safe sexual behaviour and the use of care and support services by adults. Counselling people on HIV/

Box 19: Making HIV counselling and testing work—some recommendations

In 1999, Population Council and Family Health International brought together scientists, policy-makers, health service providers, activists and community members to discuss HIV counselling and testing in Asia. The objectives were: to review relevant research and programme experiences; to debate critical issues in designing and implementing policies and programmes; and to identify priorities for operational research.

VCT as an entry point for HIV prevention and care
Evidently, many countries use HIV testing to track down and isolate PLWH. Even where informed consent, counselling and confidentiality procedures exist, many health workers are unfamiliar with them or ignore them altogether. Testing is often conducted without consent, with the results disclosed to other health workers and family members. Those who test positive often experience psychological distress and discrimination. Such abuses can be avoided by protecting the rights and needs of PLWH and developing regulatory and quality assurance procedures. Shifting the emphasis to voluntary and confidential testing can actually lead to more HIV testing. Participants concluded that counselling and testing should serve as entry points to a continuum of care, and should be designed to address the multiple needs and rights of individuals at risk or those already infected. Greater involvement of PLWH in care and support programmes can improve the quality and relevance of services and curb stigma and discrimination.

The role of VCT in the prevention of mother-to-child transmission of HIV
VCT plays a pivotal role in interventions to prevent MTCT. However, maternal counselling and consent have not always received sufficient attention and are narrowly focused on potential benefits to the newborn, neglecting the needs of the mother. Participants felt that more attention should be paid to meeting needs of mothers, especially with regard to consent, confidentiality and ongoing personal care and support. They called for further research to assess the feasibility, acceptability and cost of different approaches to PMTCT in various settings in the region.

Service delivery models
A key challenge lies in improving access to services while ensuring that they meet basic standards with respect to consent, confidentiality and quality (counselling) and validity (testing). The most promising service delivery models address a diverse set of individual and community needs. Operational research should aim at innovation, experimentation and evaluation of various service delivery models.

Implications of new technologies
Simple and rapid HIV testing would facilitate the expansion of VCT services, but in settings where inadequate attention is paid to consent and confidentiality, such tests may also increase the risk of coercion. Access to simple and rapid tests should be tightly controlled and extreme caution should be exercised in their use. Guidelines and protocols, especially for confirmatory tests, also need to be carefully developed.

Ethical and legal issues
Concern was expressed about the ethical and legal dimensions of HIV counselling and testing. An appropriate legal framework for HIV testing needs to be developed. Such laws should be based on extensive consultation (especially with PLWH organizations) and a review of legal mechanisms to protect the rights of PLWH.

Source: Family Health International 2000.

AIDS does not merely consist of stating facts and providing methods of contraception. It includes helping clients find healthier and safer ways to live. Effective counselling can help clients and counsellors explore, express, understand and accept feelings and process information in order to foster informed decision-making. This can reduce the risk of and vulnerability to STIs and HIV/AIDS.

Couple counselling, often used in high-prevalence populations, has proven effective in reducing high-risk behaviour, particularly among HIV-discordant couples.[323] Studies also indicate that men are more easily persuaded to use condoms when couples are counselled together. Community education campaigns may help to encourage reluctant men to participate in counselling.

Women in difficult relationships may seek counselling without their partners in order to have a safe place to discuss intimate issues and personal challenges in their lives. Family planning providers should be trained to recognize these potential problems and recommend individual counselling for women who may face risks or difficulties in being counselled with their partner.

Group counselling can help people identify their own problems by listening to others' experiences. Finding out what people want to talk about is the first step. Once that is discovered, opportunities for integration of HIV and STI components will arise.

Treatment and care

Comprehensive treatment and care services for people living with HIV and AIDS include diagnosis, prophylaxis and treatment of opportunistic infections (OIs), antiretroviral therapy and palliative care. Clinical treatment and care should be complemented by prevention messages, counselling and a variety of support services, such as those that provide adequate nutrition, psychological, social, and daily living support.[324] Services for the treatment and care of HIV/AIDS must be equitable, accessible, affordable, comprehensive and sustainable over the long term.

An integral aspect of the international and national commitments to universal access is access to HIV treatment for all those in need. While effective treatment for HIV/AIDS became available in 1996—with the discovery that certain combinations of three or more anti-AIDS drugs could substantially suppress the virus for sustained periods, triple antiretroviral treatment (ART) has only recently been integrated into comprehensive treatment and care for HIV/AIDS in developing countries.[325] For many years, the high costs of ARVs in combination with weak health systems led to the common belief that scaling up access to ART was unfeasible in low- and middle-income countries. This translated into a global gap in access to ART, with roughly 7% of those in need receiving ART globally in 2003. Dramatic price reductions and sustained advocacy have changed attitudes towards treatment and have increased the availability of ART in developing countries.

In response to inequalities in access to ART, WHO and UNAIDS launched a global campaign to provide three million people living with HIV/AIDS in low- and middle-income countries with ART by the end of 2005. With this ambitious plan, WHO and UNAIDS hoped to reach 50% of those in need globally as an interim target towards universal access to treatment. In the Region, the campaign targeted roughly 70 000 people in need of treatment in Cambodia, China, Papua New Guinea and Viet Nam. At the end of 2005, 1.3 million people were receiving ART globally. By 2006, roughly 24% of those in need had access to ART. Estimates from the Region suggest that by June 2006, ARVs were reaching 30% of those in need. This represented a significant increase from the roughly 8% receiving treatment in 2004. Progress was most rapid in Cambodia, where more than 70% of people in need of treatment are now receiving ART. Table 7 presents estimates of ART coverage by region.[326]

While the "3 by 5" campaign did not meet its goal of reaching three million people by 2005,

Table 7: Estimated number of people receiving and needing antiretroviral therapy and the percentage coverage in low- and middle-income countries by region, June 2006

Region	Estimated number of people receiving ARV therapy [low estimate – high estimate]	Estimated number of people needing ARV therapy	ARV coverage
Sub-Saharan Africa	1 040 000 [930 000 – 1 150 000]	4 600 000	23%
Latin America and the Caribbean	345 000 [260 000 – 430 000]	460 000	75%
East, South and South-East Asia	235 000 [180 000 – 290 000]	1 440 000	16%
Europe and Central Asia	24 000 [23 000 – 25 000]	190 000	13%
North Africa and the Middle East	4000 [3000 – 5000]	75 000	5%
Total	1 650 000 [1 400 000 – 1 900 000]	6 800 000	24%

Source: World Health Organization and Joint United Nations Programme on HIV/AIDS 2006.

significant progress was made in expanding treatment to those in need in low- and middle-income countries. This progress was matched by renewed commitment for HIV prevention, for capacity-building of health systems, and for the extension of services for long-term, chronic care. Importantly, "3 by 5" established ART as an integral component of a comprehensive approach to HIV/AIDS prevention and control in developing countries.[327] The experiences of Cambodia, China, Papua New Guinea, Thailand and Viet Nam point to the importance of political will at the national and local levels and the need for sufficient management capacity, among other factors, in rapidly scaling up access to ART.[328] The momentum built up by the "3 by 5" campaign is pushing countries towards universal access.

Universal access

Based on the experience of the "3 by 5" initiative, developing countries are increasing their political and financial commitment to scaling up access to ART. WHO recommends a public health approach to expanding the delivery of ART in developing countries, which includes a simplified and standardized approach to treatment regimes. These guidelines are found in Section 6 of this module. National plans for ART must be based on a model of chronic care, in which individual patients receive continuous follow-up treatment for the remainder of their lives, rather than the occasional acute interventions that characterize the response to most infectious diseases.[329] In addition, WHO recommends an integrated approach to service delivery and the training of health staff on the integrated management of adult illness (for more details, see Section 6, Resources).[330]

Given limited resources, only selected individuals will receive treatment and care services when ART coverage is scaled up in a phased manner. This raises issues of equity in access to treatment for vulnerable groups, which already face a disproportionately high risk of infection due to social, economic and cultural discrimination and lack of access to health services. Deep social and economic inequalities and disparities in access to health services characterize many areas in which efforts towards universal access are being implemented. Because of this, equity considerations need to figure strongly in plans to scale up access to ART. Indeed, in countries where HIV infection is concentrated within certain groups, prevention and treatment efforts need to be targeted accordingly. For countries in the Western Pacific Region with low prevalence rates, this is an opportunity to target resources effectively.

Thus, eligibility criteria for treatment may need to include biomedical as well as socioeconomic vulnerabilities. Similarly, eligibility criteria cannot discriminate against women based on their pregnancy status, or focus on women only in relation to pregnancies.[331] Broad-based commitment to establishing such eligibility

> **Box 20: Reaching the poor in Rio de Janeiro**
>
> Rio de Janeiro, the second largest city in Brazil, has 5.8 million inhabitants, of which more than a million live in slums. Since the first HIV case was registered in 1982, the number of notified infections has risen to 24 000. Most of these are concentrated in the poorest neighbourhoods. Despite having numerous hospitals and clinics in the city, access to care is constrained. Since 1992, following the national government's example, the city government has implemented a package of prevention and care services. Universal free access to triple antiretroviral treatment began in 1996.
>
> To improve access to services, a continuously updated training programme for health workers was launched. Today, staff at 51 health facilities, including university hospitals and primary care units, provide antiretroviral drugs to more than 19 000 HIV/AIDS patients in all areas. More than half of all patients are followed in primary care units where tuberculosis treatment, antenatal care and other health programmes are also in place.
>
> Along with training, several projects for vulnerable populations were started in partnership with NGOs, with financial support from the Ministry of Health. A total of 120 health units carry out prevention activities, including condom distribution, and NGOs run more than 50 projects to tackle the epidemic in specific populations.
>
> A community health workers' programme works in partnership with community-based organizations to disseminate prevention messages, bring those unaware of their infection to where they can receive help, and reduce stigma. Training and support groups to promote adherence were started in clinics, with active contribution by NGOs. So far, the evaluation of treatment adherence and drug resistance in Brazil show results similar to those in developed countries.
>
> Locally, partnership with civil society has fostered innovation. Local and national political support and recognition of HIV/AIDS as a public health problem has been critical in the fast scale-up of activities. As a result of this multisectoral effort, AIDS-related deaths decreased by around 70% in Rio de Janeiro. A drop in hospital admissions and a rise in outpatient clinic visits testify to the widespread improvement in treating AIDS-related illness.
>
> Source: World Health Organization 2004b.

criteria may be supported through processes that expand access to treatment in a transparent and accountable manner.

Programme planners and implementers, working with communities, can take steps to reduce existing inequalities in access to treatment, including those that are gender-based. The active involvement of groups representing poor and marginalized communities is crucial, as experience in Rio de Janeiro shows (see Box 20).[332] Involving women living with HIV/AIDS in all aspects of planning and implementation can ensure that efforts to scale up access to ART respond adequately to their perspectives and needs, including through innovative strategies to reach women with ART.[333] As discussed in the sections above, experience has revealed a number of barriers to access to treatment for poor people living with HIV/AIDS. Because of this, it is increasingly clear that financing strategies that subsidize or provide ART free of charge at point of service and eliminate registration and other user fees can increase access for poor and marginalized individuals.[334] In response, WHO has advised countries to adopt a policy of free access at point-of-service delivery to HIV care and treatment, including ART.[335]

Stigma has been found to be the most significant barrier to treatment in many countries. Sustained efforts are thus required to reduce stigmatizing behaviour on the part of health service providers and the general public. In addition, counselling services that are private and confidential are needed to encourage people to seek treatment, care and support from health facilities. However, research shows that health centres in resource-poor settings often lack the facilities to offer confidential counselling services.[336]

Since women face particular vulnerabilities, their treatment needs should figure strongly in efforts to reach universal access to treatment. To date, little gender-bias in access to treatment has been recorded globally.[337] Figure 12 presents the proportion of women who are receiving ART in selected countries in the Region. To ensure that women benefit equitably from investments in ART, initiatives are required to address the barriers women face when accessing health services. For example, user fees may discourage women from accessing care more than men because women may have lower access to and control over household resources than men. As such, when devising financing schemes for ART, including eligibility for free or subsidized treatment, the gendered impact of user fees needs to be considered. Free or subsidized access to ART may disproportionately and particularly benefit women and young people.[338]

Research from various countries shows that health staff are often unaware of, and inconsiderate towards, women's particular health needs and the constraints they might face when seeking to access health services. In some instances, health staff have been found to blame women for delayed treatment-seeking.[339] Poor women have been found to be particularly sensitive to the behaviour of health staff, and might not access formal health services when they perceive health service providers to be disrespectful and insensitive to their needs.[340] Box 21 outlines a number of strategies to ensure equal access for men and women to treatment for HIV/AIDS.

Improving the responsiveness of HIV/AIDS treatment and care

A core component of scaling up access to ART is strengthening the capacity of the health system to deliver comprehensive treatment and care services for HIV/AIDS. This may be of particular concern

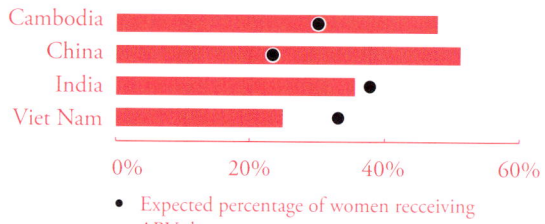

Figure 12: Women as a percentage of all adults receiving antiretroviral therapy in selected countries, actual verses expected percentages, 2005

Source: Joint United Nations Programme on HIV/AIDS and World Health Organization, 2006a.

in underserved areas, where the quality of health care tends to be substandard. Improving a number of elements of health systems are thus required to reach the target of universal access for poor and marginalized communities.

An absolute shortage of health workers with adequate skills in HIV/AIDS prevention, treatment and care is only one of many serious challenges to meeting the human resource needs for universal access to treatment and care. Other challenges include the maldistribution of workers and tasks; migration of health workers; low retention of trained personnel in their positions and/or the country where they are trained; unfavourable working conditions and occupational safety; stigma attached to working on HIV/AIDS; and the impact of HIV/AIDS on staff themselves. Finally, although a well-trained workforce is an essential prerequisite to high-quality health care, quality is also determined by the organization of the health care system in which the workforce operates.[341] Efforts are thus needed to tackle the shortage and maldistribution of human resources for health and the generally low remuneration for health staff, especially in underserved areas, that can result in poor quality services, absenteeism and many vacancies. The impact of HIV/AIDS on the workforce is exacerbating an already difficult situation.[342] A number of innovative strategies have been documented in this context. In several countries, private companies have successfully delivered ART beyond the workplace to neighbouring communities. Providing the existing pool of

> **Box 21: Ensuring equal access for women and men**
>
> In most countries, gender relations are characterized by an unequal balance of power between women and men, with women having fewer legal rights and lower access to education, training, income-generating activities, property and health services. These factors affect their ability to protect themselves from HIV as well as their access to health knowledge, treatment and care. Ideally, health interventions will not only recognize and respond to the existing situation, but promote transformative approaches that challenge unequal gender roles and relations.
>
> The following are crucial considerations in the design of gender-sensitive treatment programmes.
>
> **Access to information**. Providing information about the availability and benefits of antiretroviral treatment ("treatment literacy") is vital to generating and sustaining demand. The avenues (such as radio, drama and peer groups) used to reach people with information, and the messages given, may be different for women and men.
>
> **Access to services**. Services need to tackle the gender-specific barriers to access that women face relative to men: economic, cultural, opportunity cost (distance, timing of services and waiting time may make the service inaccessible to women), stigma and discrimination, and quality of care. Involving people in the design of services can help identify these barriers, improve the design of services and involve communities in the provision of support.
>
> **Entry points for antiretroviral treatment**. While antenatal services constitute an obvious entry point for identifying women in need of treatment, outreach to women with HIV who are not pregnant, particularly young women, is necessary.
>
> **Barriers to testing and counselling**. The decision to seek testing is influenced by risk perception. Many married women who are monogamous and faithful may not feel themselves to be at risk. Women often fear the negative outcomes of testing, such as stigma, discrimination, increased violence or abandonment.
>
> **Barriers to disclosure**. Women's justifiable fears of the consequences of disclosure, such as violence and rejection, need to be tackled. These appear to be more common when a woman is tested in front of her partner. Couple counselling and testing, mediated disclosure by a trained counsellor, and education of communities and family members can all help to reduce stigma and discrimination against women who test positive. Women's right to confidentiality should be respected.
>
> **Monitoring and follow-up**. Monitoring should be ongoing in order to identify who is being reached and who is not, and to make the necessary adjustments. Countries should be encouraged to set specific targets for women, based on local epidemiology.
>
> **Training of providers**. Integrating gender considerations into treatment initiatives is an opportunity to focus on gender-based violence and other barriers.
>
> Source: World Health Organization 2004b.

community health workers, medical assistance and other community-based health personnel with the necessary knowledge and skills to manage treatment for people with HIV/AIDS can improve the delivery of ART in poor and remote communities. Care needs to be taken, however, to ensure that these health care workers receive adequate training and support.[343]

Building the capacity of health care workers can also enable the extension of ART into underserved areas. Training is required to improve the ability of health care workers to deliver an integrated approach to ART, care and prevention. Investing in efforts to strengthen providers' motivation, reduce AIDS stigma in the health sector, improve working conditions and encourage positive attitudes toward providing antiretroviral therapy and care can also improve the quality of care for PLWH. WHO and International Labour Organization (ILO) have developed new guidelines to protect the safety of health workers involved in HIV/AIDS. The guidelines include wide-ranging and practical approaches to protection, training, screening, treatment, confidentiality, prevention, the minimizing of occupational risk, and the care and support of health care providers.[344]

Adherence to antiretroviral therapy

Ensuring adherence to treatment is key to preventing drug resistance and to ensuring the effectiveness of ARV regimens. Adherence levels of at least 95% are required to ensure positive treatment outcomes and prevent the rise of drug resistance.[345] Strategies to support improved adherence among poor men and women might include outreach and other innovative efforts that bring treatment services closer to poor households and communities. This can reduce transportation costs and overcome difficulties associated with limited or irregular transportation in remote and small island communities. Increasing the coverage of treatment centres would likewise reduce transportation costs. Scheduling clinic hours that are convenient for HIV patients, such as in the early morning or evening for those who work during the day, as well as reducing waiting times can decrease the opportunity costs associated with clinical visits and securing ARV refills. Support to ensure that poor patients have access to adequate food, particularly during the first months of treatment, may also improve adherence to treatment.

Culturally appropriate adherence support should be developed in order to address the special problems associated with pregnant and postpartum women. Adherence may be more difficult in pregnant women and immediately postpartum women than in non-pregnant individuals. Pregnancy-associated morning sickness and gastrointestinal upset may complicate ART and the situation may be exacerbated by ARV-associated side-effects or concern about the potential effects of drugs on the foetus. In the postpartum period, physical changes and the demands of caring for a newborn infant may compromise maternal drug adherence.

In general, little evidence is available on the adherence to treatment by men as compared with women in developing countries. Gender was not identified as a significant factor in a review of available evidence on adherence to treatment.[346] A study in Botswana reported that adherence to treatment was similar among men and women. However, qualitative research carried out during the same study revealed that acceptance of HIV status, disclosure and gender influenced adherence to treatment. That is, women were more likely than men to accept their HIV status and thus more likely than men to seek treatment for HIV. The study points to the need for further research into these issues.

Home-based care

The majority of people living with AIDS in the developing world are cared for at home by family members. Home-based care encompasses the care and support provided within the home and external support provided to the HIV patient and household members by community health workers and volunteers; visiting nurses and social workers may also play a role.[347] NGOs, church groups and community organizations often participate actively in home care initiatives. Experience shows that, to be effective, support for home-based care should include medical treatment and care, training and basic medical supplies for caregivers, psychosocial counselling, support for household work and income-generating activities.[348] However, given the diversity of households affected by HIV/AIDS, a needs assessment is a critical first step when planning a support programme.

The economic costs associated with caring for PLWH at home can strain the already limited resources of poor households and may lead to further impoverishment in the long run. In most countries, gender roles determine how the burden of caring for someone with HIV/AIDS will be distributed among household members. The burden of home care tends to fall on women and girls. While this work is often cast as voluntary or free labour, the responsibility to care for the sick can actually impose high opportunity costs, forcing women to leave paid employment or cut back on agricultural work and obliging girls to drop out of school. In response, home care programmes need to be tailored to meet the needs of poor households and to benefit women. In addition, men must be encouraged to increase their participation in caregiving and supported in doing so. A more equal distribution of duties between men and women can reduce the disproportionate burden on women and girls and may also lead increased visibility and valuation of caregiving within households.

Monitoring and evaluation of poverty/equity and gender in HIV/AIDS

Despite the growing recognition of ongoing and often increasing health inequities both in developing and developed countries, health information systems have, to date, been weak in yielding information needed to assess and address health inequities. The challenge is to determine the information needs for addressing health inequities; to shape health information systems to meet those needs; to promote sensitization to equity issues; and to develop the skills required to use information for effective planning and policy-making.[349]

In addition to increasing the availability of various data sources, improvements need to be made in the equity-relevant information included. To assess health equity adequately, equity indicators must be constructed. This requires a health measure (or measure of determinant of health) and an equity stratifier (such as a measure of socioeconomic position, sex, age, ethnicity/race, and/or geographical position), as well as the ability to disaggregate information according to these stratifiers.

This can be accomplished either by ensuring that appropriate equity stratifiers and health measures are available in each data source, or by creating mechanisms to link records between data sources. For example, effective links can be created by including a unique identifier or geographical code in a variety of data sources. The Health Metrics Network has begun work on constructing equity indicators and creating mechanisms to link records between data sources.[350]

An evaluation tool to assess the poverty-responsiveness and gender-sensitivity of HIV/AIDS programmes is given in Box 30 (see Section 6, Tools). Senior and local health care administrators and health care practitioners may review these evaluation questions and revise, adapt or include other items for evaluation that reflect their local situations. Responses to this evaluation should then be reported to senior administration together with recommendations for action. Senior administration, together with local health care administrators, practitioners and PLWH should then develop a plan of action to address the issues identified as requiring further attention. It is important to remember that this evaluation tool is to be used as a foundation for further action to promote poverty and gender-sensitive programmes and services for PLWH.

Research

Continual research is required to create more effective strategies in the response to AIDS. Collecting and sharing evidence on innovative HIV prevention efforts that have proven to be effective are key in halting the spread of the epidemic. Additional clinical research is required to generate new antiretroviral drugs and therapeutic strategies.[351] Operational research to improve the accessibility and availability of HIV care and treatment has, until now, been largely neglected by both researchers and funding organizations. To discover and improve methods of scaling up access to treatment, economic analysis must be coupled with clinical data provided by longitudinal follow-up of patients in resource-poor settings. It is important to identify the factors that affect efforts to increase access to treatment, particularly in the context of health services and with regards to health policy. The effect of different financing arrangements of HIV treatment and care on treatment adherence, the development of drug resistance, and final treatment outcomes likewise need to be significant topics of study. Efforts are likewise required to address gender bias in HIV/AIDS research, such as that discussed above. In addition to including women in clinical trials and other studies to improve the gender responsiveness of HIV/AIDS prevention, treatment and care, research methodologies need to be scrutinised to ensure that men and women's biological and gender-related vulnerabilities are captured. Finally, research to design a safe and effective preventive vaccine remains the best hope for the long-term prevention and control of HIV/AIDS. Box 22 presents some examples of international research efforts.

Box 22: Some international research efforts

Over time, the prevalence of HIV infection has fallen among pregnant women in urban areas of **Uganda**. Research suggests that this was due to increased condom use, delay in the onset of sexual intercourse, and/or a reduction in the number of sexual partners. Combining evidence on HIV prevalence and sexual behaviour were shown to contribute greatly to the success of HIV prevention programmes.[352]

In **Abidjan**, **Cote d'Ivoire**, the prevalence of HIV infection in female sex workers fell from 89% to 32% between 1991 and 1998. This decline was attributed to an increase in condom use. In 1992, 20% of sex workers used condoms in their most recent working day, while in 1998, this number rose to 78%. The report suggested that sustained prevention efforts and the promotion of condom use built around local initiatives were central to this success.

Analysis of a youth-targeted social marketing campaign in **Cameroon** was undertaken to assess the effectiveness of the programme to promote sexual and reproductive health among young people aged 13–22 years of age. Among other factors, the results of the study demonstrated the importance of involving young people in the design of the programme. Incorporating a sound understanding of the sexual health concerns of men and addressing the stigma associated with condom use were likely found to be pivotal to the effectiveness of the programme.

Sources: Ashford 2000; Agha 2000; Van Rossem and Meekers 2000.

5. Facilitator's notes

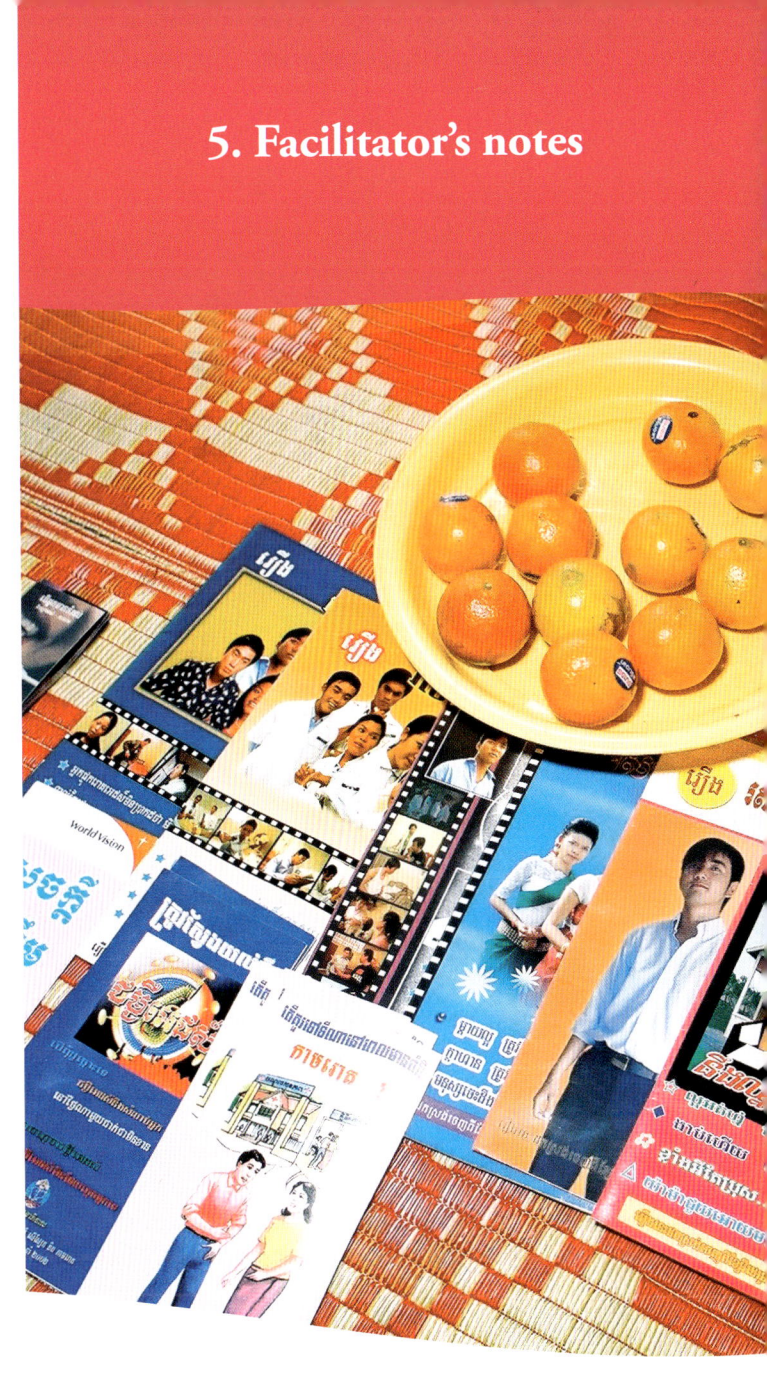

5. Facilitator's notes

These notes are provided to support facilitators as they work with learners on integrating poverty and gender issues into specific health topics. Facilitators are recommended to refer to Section 5 of the foundational modules of this Sourcebook, dealing respectively with poverty and gender, which contain additional notes on the target audience, role of the facilitator and suggested methodologies for learning sessions and for evaluation.

The learning sessions and exercises that follow are practical and oriented toward "active learning". That is, they are designed to promote group discussion and presentation in analysing HIV/AIDS in terms of gender and poverty. The time required for all learning sessions is approximately 16 hours.

Expected learning outcomes

Upon completion of the module, participants will be able to:
- demonstrate an understanding of HIV/AIDS, including the distribution and characteristics of HIV/AIDS epidemics;
- demonstrate an understanding of WHAT the links are between poverty, gender and HIV/AIDS;
- explain WHY it is important for health professionals to address poverty and gender concerns in HIV/AIDS, from efficiency, equity and human rights perspectives;
- indicate HOW health professionals and the health care system as a whole can address poverty and gender concerns in HIV/AIDS;
- demonstrate an understanding of international and national policies and guidelines, programme planning and financing, and service delivery;
- demonstrate an awareness of good practice interventions at the health facility, community and policy levels; and
- demonstrate familiarity with some tools, resources and references available to health professionals in dealing with HIV/AIDS.

Activity 1: Declarations on poverty and gender in HIV/AIDS

Objective: To begin a discussion about poverty and gender as they relate to HIV/AIDS

Time required: 3 hours

Pre-reading: Section 2: poverty, gender and HIV/AIDS

Suggested exercise

Step 1. Brainstorming session: Poverty and HIV/AIDS

Process: Write "Poverty and HIV/AIDS" at the top of a flip chart. Ask participants how poverty impacts upon HIV/AIDS and how poverty is impacted by HIV/AIDS. Write all the responses on the flip chart. Put the same title at the top of each new sheet. Hang the completed flip chart papers around the room.

Notes to the facilitator

Be sure the group first identifies how poverty increases the probability of HIV infection and progression to AIDS-related morbidity and mortality. Issues that should be identified include those related to:
- increased vulnerability to HIV/AIDS
- restricted choice of safe economic activities
- health-seeking behaviours and access to health care
- economic migration
- lower levels of education
- indirect relationship between poverty and HIV/AIDS (e.g. lower nutritional status)
- ethnic minorities
- poor urban and rural settings
- vulnerable youth and children
- vulnerable older people

Then, ask the participants to identify how HIV/AIDS induces or deepens poverty. Issues that should be identified include those related to:

- reduction in national income
- loss of social capital
- loss of productivity
- job loss, stigma and discrimination
- farming, food insecurity and loss of land
- education, poverty and HIV/AIDS
- catastrophic costs of care
- increased dependency ratio
- opportunity costs of care
- indirect costs of care (e.g. additional costs for food, orphan care, funerals, etc.)

Step 2. Brainstorming session: Gender and HIV/AIDS

Process: Write "Gender and HIV/AIDS" at the top of a flip chart. Ask participants to identify the links between gender and HIV/AIDS. Be sure that the participants speak separately about girls/women and boys/men. Write their responses on the flip chart paper. If more pages are needed, write the title at the top of each new piece of paper. Hang the completed papers around the room.

Notes to the facilitator

Part 1: Vulnerability of women and girls

Make sure participants identify the following issues:
- gender norms
- lack of education
- lack of access to services and resources
- sexual customs and norms
- sexual cleansing
- unequal control in gender relationships
- gender-based violence
- social disruption and religious and ethnic intolerance
- lack of economic opportunities
- HIV and prostitution
- stigma and discrimination
- gender bias in HIV/AIDS prevention, treatment and research
- the role of girls and women in family care-giving and orphan care
- legal obstacles and lack of political will

Part 2: Vulnerability of men and boys

Make sure participants identify the following issues:
- lack of access to information and education
- lack of access to services and resources
- multiple sex partners
- risk-taking behaviours
- men who have sex with men
- male sex workers
- prisons and HIV/AIDS
- military and HIV/AIDS

Step 3. Determining the major issues: poverty and HIV/AIDS

Process: Return to the flip chart papers on which are written the issues related to poverty and HIV/AIDS. Ask the participants to determine the major issues identified during the brainstorming session on poverty and HIV/AIDS. In order to help with this exercise, ask the participants to cluster issues that could be put under one heading. For example, the group might have identified lack of money for food, drugs or medical treatment. This might be clustered into "lack of access to necessary resources". The names for the clusters can be determined by the participants, or you might choose to help the group with naming each cluster. Go through each issue identified during the brainstorming session and determine the appropriate cluster. Use this time to discuss further the issues identified in the brainstorming session. This can be quite a complex process. However, it helps participants identify the major issues related to poverty and HIV/AIDS. Write the larger cluster titles on a separate piece of flip chart paper and stick on the wall.

Step 4. Determining the major issues: gender and HIV/AIDS

Process: Continue the same clustering exercise as above, focusing on gender and HIV/AIDS. Remind the participants to include women, girls, boys and men in their clustering. The cluster titles do not have to identify whether they apply to men or women; however, ask questions that determine if a particular cluster affects only men or women, or is relevant to both sexes. You will now end up with two (or perhaps more) flip chart pages that identify the clusters associated with poverty and gender in relation to HIV/AIDS.

Step 5. Writing a declaration on poverty and HIV/AIDS

Process: Return to the flip chart page(s) with the clusters associated with poverty and HIV/AIDS. Using these cluster titles, work with participants to come up with a declaration against poverty and HIV/AIDS. Write the declaration on another flip chart paper. This declaration does not have to be "word perfect"; rather it is a joint effort by the participants to declare their intentions about addressing poverty and HIV/AIDS. To that end, be sure the participants use strong verbs such as advocate, lobby, ensure, reduce, etc. The overall intention of this exercise is to have the participants see themselves as activists in addressing poverty and HIV/AIDS.

Step 6. Writing a declaration on gender and HIV/AIDS

Process: Repeat the exercise above (Step 5). This time, however, use the clusters associated with gender and HIV/AIDS.

Activity 2: Influencing change

Objective: To engage in influencing policy formation and practices within government in relation to poverty, gender and HIV/AIDS

Time allotted: 2 hours

Pre-reading: Section 3 of the module on HIV/AIDS

Suggested exercise

Step 1. Setting the activity

Process: Divide the participants into three groups. Assign each group one of the three sections found in Section 3 of this module containing the rationales for addressing poverty and gender issues in HIV/AIDS: (1) efficiency, (2) equity, and (3) human rights. That is, one group will receive the section on efficiency, the second group, the section on equity and the final group will receive the section on human rights. Explain to the groups that, as senior health administrators for their district, they have been asked to present the issues related to gender and poverty in relation to HIV/AIDS to a newly formed National AIDS Committee. Each group of senior administrators has been asked to focus on one aspect of this challenge: efficiency, equity and human rights.

Ask each group to read through the issues outlined in their particular section. Explain that they have 30 minutes to prepare a statement to be presented to the National AIDS Committee. Ask one person (or perhaps a couple of people) per group to volunteer to present the group's statements to the National AIDS Committee. The rest of the participants will act as committee members.

Step 2. Presentation to committee and general discussion

Process: Each group has 5 minutes to present their case to the National AIDS Committee (the other participants). Following each presentation, the committee members have 10 minutes to ask why these particular issues are more important than other pressing issues. The purpose of this exercise is to generate discussion between the committee members (the participants) and the senior administrators making the presentation (the presenting group). Explain to the "members" that, as the committee, they have to choose between a series of very important options; therefore, they should ask searching questions to ascertain whether these issues warrant special attention. The "senior administrators" (the presenting group) must be prepared to answer these questions and convince the committee that these policies need to be put into practice.

Repeat this exercise two more times so that each group of "senior administrators" can present and argue its case and answer the searching questions posed by the National AIDS Committee (the rest of the participants).

Step 3. Debriefing

Process: Bring the participants together to debrief. Questions you might pose to the group include:
- How did it feel to present a case to a committee, knowing that they might choose only some of the options (if any) you proposed?
- How did it feel to speak out about an important issue? (Prompts might include: Did you feel powerful? Powerless? Frustrated?)
- Do you think that health professionals can influence policy formation and practice?
- Can you see yourself taking on such a role? If yes, why? If not, why not?

Activity 3: Case study problem-solving exercise

Objective: To develop problem-solving abilities related to gender, poverty and HIV/AIDS

Time allotted: 2 hours

Pre-reading: Section 2 of the module on HIV/AIDS

Step 1. Group discussion of case studies

Process: Divide the class into five groups. Distribute case scenarios to the groups. Ask one group member to take notes of the discussion and be prepared to report back to the larger group at the end of the group session.

Case study 1: You are working in an antenatal care (ANC) centre where the policy is to encourage women to be tested for HIV as part of their antenatal screening. What would be your immediate considerations and how would you approach HIV testing with the women who visit your clinic?

Notes to the facilitator: The following issues should be identified and discussed by the group as part of the problem-solving exercise:
- voluntary counselling (making sure it is really *voluntary*);
- confidentiality;
- knowledge about the possible repercussions of disclosure of HIV status (e.g. abandonment, violence, abuse, rejection); and
- effective counselling (pre- and post-test and continued psychosocial support).

Case study 2: A woman comes to your hospital complaining of pain in her arm. You know that she is pregnant and has tested positive for HIV. When you examine her arm you see considerable bruising and swelling. You ask her how she injured her arm and she is evasive. What issues would be going through your mind? How would you approach this woman? Remember, you do not know the cause of this injury. What might be your course of action?

Notes to the facilitator: The following issues, approaches and course of action should be identified and discussed by the group as part of the problem-solving exercise:
1. **Issue:** possible partner abuse and family rejection.
2. Approaches:
   - Be tentative and sensitive to the woman's vulnerability.
     - Provide a case example (using anonymity) to let the woman know you are aware of the risks of disclosure.
3. Course of action:
   - Wait for the woman to explain her condition. If she does not, let the woman know you will be able to help her at a future time, should she wish to see you.
   - Make another appointment for the woman.
   - Assure her that you will help her when she is ready.

Case study 3: You are a health administrator in a district with a high incidence and prevalence of HIV/AIDS. Most of the population lives in poverty and their access to health care is limited. As an administrator, you have been asked to develop a policy for improving access to health care for people living in absolute poverty. The government has agreed to provide funds to assist the destitute with access to essential health care. How would you go about developing this policy? Who should be involved in these policy decisions?

Notes to the facilitator: The following issues should be identified and discussed by the group as part of the problem-solving exercise:
- How would policy guidelines for destitute allowance be developed?
- Who would be responsible for this development?
- How would you ensure access to health care for people in absolute poverty?
- What kind of monitoring system would you develop to deliver the programme and be accountable to government?
- Who should be involved in policy development: government representatives, PLWH, destitute people, financial administrators, health care workers?

Case study 4: You have noticed that many young people in your community are engaged in high-risk behaviours such as drinking alcohol and engaging in unprotected sexual intercourse. Most of these young people are still students. As a health professional, what can you do to address this problem? What might be some barriers to working with young people? What might be some of the strengths in working with young people? Who would you work with to ensure young people are involved in prevention messages?

Notes to the facilitator: The following issues should be identified and discussed by the group as part of the problem-solving exercise:
- involve young people in prevention messages and other prevention strategies;
- use peer support;
- involve young people in media messages;
- work with teachers, school administrators and other educators;
- access community services and resources that focus on young people;
- barriers: young people are risk-averse;
- natural risk-taking behaviours of young people;
- peer pressure; and
- social norms and expectations of young people.

Case study 5: A young boy comes to the health centre with urethral discharge. He is very shy and will not discuss his sexual history. He is diagnosed with an STI. As a health professional, what are your concerns? How might you approach this situation?

Notes to the facilitator: The following concerns and approaches should be identified and discussed by the group as part of the problem-solving exercise:
1. Concerns:
   - possible exposure to HIV infection
   - difficult to talk to (shy)
   - lack of knowledge of STI transmission
   - possible lack of knowledge about anatomy and transmission of infection.
2. Approaches:
   - Give examples (with anonymity) to help the youth understand that others have had a similar problem.
   - Encourage the boy to visit a peer support group.
   - Access peer education.
   - Urge the school to provide sex education including lessons on STI and HIV transmission.
   - Suggest the youth return for further testing of STI and possible VCT for HIV.

Step 2. Debriefing on the case studies

Process: Call the participants back together. Ask the spokesperson from each group to explain the case study and then discuss their areas of concern and strategies for action. Then, ask the whole class to comment on the concerns and actions proposed by the group. Explain that there are no "right" or "wrong" concerns or strategies for action. Instead, as the entire class engages in this problem-solving process, more ideas and strategies will come to light.

Activity 4: Planning poverty- and gender-sensitive HIV/AIDS programmes

Objective: To plan an HIV/AIDS programme that focuses on the needs of the poor, as well as vulnerable women, girls, boys and men.

Time allotted: 2 hours

Pre-reading: Sections 2 and 4 of the HIV/AIDS module

Step 1. Setting the activity

Process: Divide the participants into five groups. Make sure the group composition is different from previous exercises. That is, make sure participants work with different people throughout the workshop. Give each group copies of relevant tools, checklists, examples and evaluations for incorporating poverty and gender sensitivity into HIV/AIDS programmes and services. Each group will develop a plan that will be presented by a volunteer spokesperson to other members of the class.

Group 1: Advise this group to develop a plan of action for an HIV/AIDS programme. The group should follow the checklist, "Mobilizing resources for HIV/AIDS programmes" (Box 8). Ask them to consider the following three questions as they develop their action plan:
1. What issues require the most attention?
2. Why are these issues important?
3. How would you go about developing an HIV/AIDS programme with these issues in mind?

Group 2: Ask this group to develop an HIV/AIDS prevention programme. They should use the checklist, "Developing effective HIV/AIDS prevention programmes" (Box 13), for this exercise. Ask them to use the following questions as their guide:
1. What are the issues of poverty that might affect this programme?
2. What gender-sensitive issues should be considered in developing this programme?

Group 3: Explain to this group that they hold middle-management positions in a local hospital. Senior administration has asked all district health facilities to develop a poverty- and gender-sensitive HIV/AIDS awareness programme for health care staff. As administrators of the hospital, the group must develop an HIV/AIDS awareness programme for the staff. This group should use the "HIV/AIDS and gender and poverty sensitivity in health care services" checklist (Box 23) to help develop this programme.

Group 4: This group is to help a local VCT service become more responsive to poverty and gender issues. Direct the group to use the section entitled "Poverty- and gender-sensitive voluntary counselling and testing (VCT)" as a guide to this service development. The report, *Current issues in HIV counselling and testing in South and Southeast Asia* by Family Health International, may also help guide Group 4 members. Write on a piece of paper the following questions to guide this group:
1. How would you evaluate the level of poverty and gender sensitivity that exists at the VCT service?
2. How would you begin to help VCT staff become more responsive to poverty and gender issues in their VCT service?
3. What are the most pressing issues that need to be incorporated into the VCT service? How would you prioritize the issues?
4. How can you encourage VCT staff to place importance on these prioritized issues?
5. What plan of action would you leave with VCT staff to encourage more poverty and gender sensitivity in their VCT service?

Group 5: A local antenatal care clinic has recently developed a PMTCT programme. However, clinic staff explain that the uptake of VCT is lower than expected, which is affecting the uptake of PMTCT. Group 5 has been asked to consult with the ANC clinic staff to determine why this might be the case. Using the checklist, "Gender-sensitive PMTCT programmes" (Box 24) as your guide, work with the staff to incorporate some of the most important poverty- and gender-related issues into their service. You

Facilitator's notes

are asked to leave a plan of action for the ANC clinic staff.

Step 2. Activity: Presentation of plans and debriefing

Process: Ask each group to present its plan to the class. Questions and discussion may follow each presentation.

Notes to the facilitator: Be sure to direct each group to the appropriate checklists and case studies. As the facilitator, you must ensure that each presentation and debriefing session provides opportunities for critique and for the identification of contentious issues. To encourage critique, consider asking the following questions to each group:
1. What are the most significant issues of this plan?
2. Should other issues have been included?
3. What would you do if programme staff appear disinterested in this programme?
4. What would you do if staff dismiss your concerns about women's vulnerability?
5. How would you approach staff who appear to discriminate against people who live with HIV, who are poor or who live on the margins of society?

At the end of the presentation and debriefing session, take 10 minutes to summarize the work of the groups and draw together the main issues that have been identified.

Workshop evaluation

Time allotted: 20 minutes

Please respond to the following questions related to the workshop by circling the number that best corresponds with your degree of learning. The scale is rated as follows:
1 = not at all   2 = somewhat   3 = well
4 = very well   5 = extremely well

1. How well do you believe you now understand the issues of poverty in relation to HIV/AIDS?
   1   2   3   4   5
2. How well do you believe you now understand the issues of women and girls' vulnerability to HIV/AIDS?
   1   2   3   4   5
3. How well do you believe you now understand the issues of men and boys' vulnerability to HIV/AIDS?
   1   2   3   4   5
4. How useful were the tools for practice?
   1   2   3   4   5
5. How well did the learning activities promote your learning?
   1   2   3   4   5
6. How well did the facilitator promote your learning?
   1   2   3   4   5

Please answer the following questions in the space provided:

1. Which aspect of the course/workshop did you find the most helpful?
2. Which aspect of the course/workshop did you find the least helpful?
3. Which aspects, if any, required more in-depth coverage?
4. Do you think this course will affect your future practice as a health professional? If yes, in what way? If not, why not?
5. What are your recommendations for future workshops on poverty, gender and HIV/AIDS?
6. Would you recommend this course/workshop to a colleague? If yes, why? If not, why not?
7. Do you have any additional comments?

6. Tools, resources and references

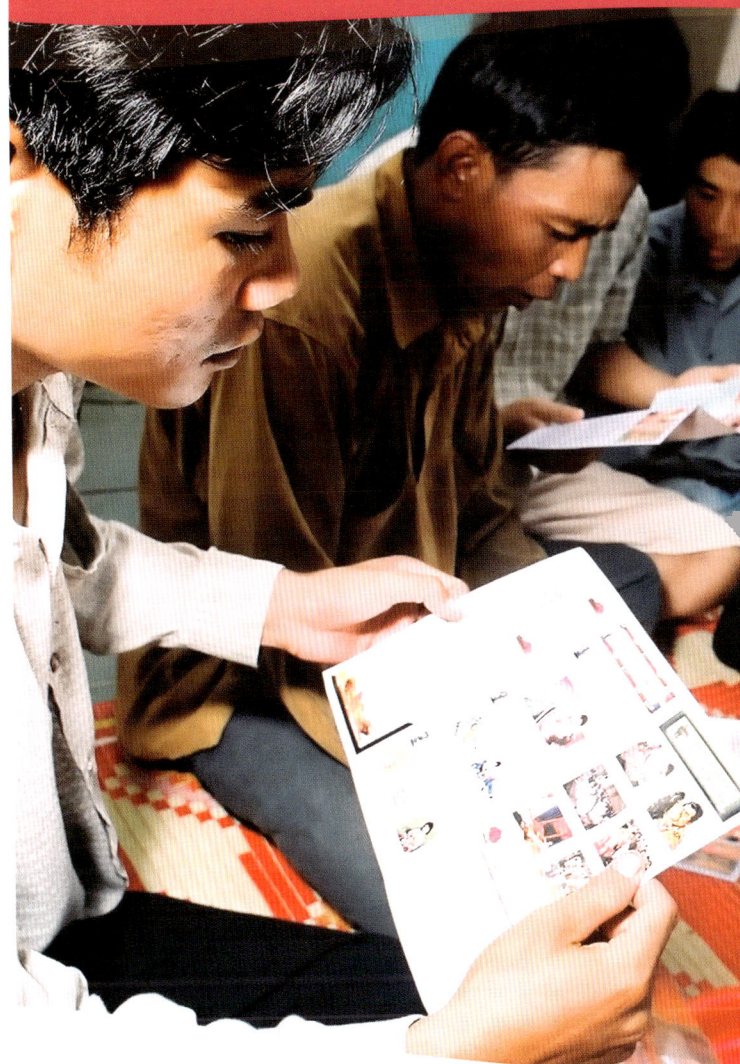

6. Tools, resources and references

Tools

This section provides guidelines, frameworks for action, and case examples to address poverty, gender and HIV/AIDS. It includes tools, checklists, protocols and evaluation methods that health practitioners and administrators can use in their daily practice.

Box 23: HIV/AIDS and gender- and poverty-sensitivity in health care services

- Develop protocols and guidelines to ensure that poor people with HIV/AIDS have equal access to health care services. Develop funding mechanisms that make it possible for poor people living with HIV to have free access to necessary care, support and treatment.
- Develop protocols and guidelines to ensure that ethnic minorities (particularly vulnerable women and girls) have equal access to health care services.
- Develop monitoring mechanisms to review the practice of providing equal access to health care for the poor, vulnerable and marginalized populations living with HIV/AIDS.
- Develop guidelines for health service providers to follow to promote sociocultural sensitivity for women and girls, as well as men and boys, living with HIV/AIDS.
- Provide health service providers with IEC materials and in-service education to increase their awareness of and sensitivity to stigma, denial, discrimination and the consequences of these issues on people affected and infected with HIV/AIDS.
- Provide health service providers with IEC materials and in-service education to increase their knowledge of the biological vulnerability of women and girls to HIV/AIDS.
- Develop treatment protocols that are specifically designed for women and girls living with HIV/AIDS.
- Develop protocols and guidelines for PMTCT, including ARV therapy and infant feeding guidelines.
- Provide health service providers with IEC materials and in-service education to increase their knowledge of and sensitivity to HIV/AIDS in older people.

Box 24: Checklist: Gender-sensitive PMTCT programmes

- Are men made to feel welcome at antenatal care clinics and MCH facilities? If not, how could they be made to feel more comfortable?
- Do marginalized women (e.g. sex workers, refugees, IDUs) have equal access to VCT and PMTCT services?
- Are partners encouraged to access VCT?
- Is "shared confidentiality" of HIV status encouraged? If so, how can you address the potential for violence, rejection, discrimination and stigma against women, which are often associated with shared confidentiality?
- Are women's reproductive rights, including the right to pregnancy termination, respected?
- Is ART available for HIV-infected pregnant women? If so, do these treatments only prevent mother-to-child transmission or do they also treat the infected woman and her partner?
- What are the infant feeding policies for HIV-infected women? Do both partners have an opportunity to choose infant feeding options? If bottle-feeding is chosen, what precautions can be put in place to avoid violence, stigma, discrimination and rejection of the woman and family?

Box 25: Activities for poverty- and gender-sensitive VCT programmes

- Provide in-service training for health care providers on VCT.
- Provide in-service education sessions for health care providers to increase their awareness of and sensitivity to issues of stigma, denial, discrimination and the consequences of this on people affected by and infected with HIV/AIDS.
- Ensure that VCT is free or affordable for people living in poverty.
- Provide VCT services (or have easy access to VCT) in STI treatment centres, MCH and PHC facilities, hospitals, and other health-related facilities.
- Encourage couple involvement in VCT.
- Provide space for confidential counselling.
- Provide VCT in antenatal clinics as a first step in PMTCT.
- Ensure adequate supervision of VCT services using quality assurance methods.
- Provide HIV test kits, gloves, antiseptics, syringes, needles, vacutainers, lancets and other laboratory equipment.
- Train laboratory technicians in HIV testing and fund laboratory quality assurance.
- Promote VCT awareness, education and support within the community, particularly as they relates to poverty and gender sensitivity.
- Conduct formative research on acceptability, demand creation and consequences of VCT within the community, paying particular attention to poverty and gender sensitivity and HIV/AIDS.
- Provide family planning services and offer referrals for related services in VCT centres.
- Link VCT services with other support services (including poverty- and gender-sensitive services) in the community through referral partnerships.

Adapted from Preble, Piwoz EG. 2002.

Box 27: Expected achievements of an HIV/AIDS prevention programme

- Raise awareness of vulnerability, particularly for women and girls.
- Promote cultural, religious and social awareness of HIV/AIDS programmes.
- Raise awareness of sex and sexuality among boys and girls, men and women.
- Promote VCT and PMTCT.
- Encourage peer support and education (youth groups for boys and girls, women's groups, street children, refugees, etc.).
- Involve PLWH and family members in HIV-prevention strategies.
- Facilitate empowerment (particularly empowerment of women, girls and boys).
- Consolidate resources (e.g. counselling, education, family planning, continuum of care).
- Forge partnerships between governments, policy-makers, law enforcement, health and social service agencies, NGOs, etc.
- Challenge HIV/AIDS denial.
- Combat violence, stigma, discrimination and rejection, particularly as they relate to women and girls.
- Ensure universal precaution practices.
- Build on the success of other HIV/AIDS prevention programmes.
- Respect human rights.

Box 28: Twelve statements from the International Community of Women Living with HIV/AIDS

1. Encouragement and support for the development of self-help groups and networks.
2. The media to realistically portray us, not to stigmatize us.
3. Accessible and affordable health care (conventional and complementary) and research into how the virus affects women.
4. Funding for services to lessen our isolation and meet our basic needs. All funds directed to us need to be supervised to make sure we receive them.
5. The right to be respected and supported in our choices about reproduction, including the right to have, or not to have, children.
6. Recognition of the right of our children and orphans to be cared for and of the importance of our role as parents.
7. Education and training of health care providers and the community about women's risk and our needs. Up-to-date and accurate information about all the issues for women living with HIV/AIDS should be easily and freely available.
8. Recognition of the fundamental human rights of all women living with HIV/AIDS, particularly women in prison, drug users and sex workers. These fundamental rights should include employment, travel without restriction and housing.
9. Research into female infectivity, including woman-to-woman transmission, and recognition of and support for lesbians living with HIV/AIDS.
10. Decision-making power and consultation at all levels of policy and programmes affecting us.
11. Economic support for women living with HIV/AIDS in developing countries to help them to be self-sufficient and independent.
12. Any definition of AIDS to include symptoms and clinical manifestations specific to women.

Source: BRIDGE 2002.

Box 29: Women and HIV/AIDS: The Barcelona Bill of Rights

As we enter the third decade of HIV/AIDS, women, especially the young and the poor, are the most affected. Because gender neutrality fuels the HIV/AIDS pandemic, it is imperative that women and girls speak out, set priorities for action and lead the global response to the crisis. Therefore, women and girls from around the world unite and urge all governments, organizations, agencies, donors, communities and individuals to make our rights a reality. Women and girls have the right:

- to live with dignity and equality;
- to bodily integrity;
- to health and health care, including treatment;
- to safety, security and freedom from fear of physical and sexual violence throughout their lives;
- to be free from stigma, discrimination, blame and denial;
- to their human rights regardless of sexual orientation;
- to sexual autonomy and sexual pleasure;
- to equity in their families;
- to education and information;
- to economic independence.

These fundamental rights shall include, but not be limited to, the right:
- to support and care which meets their particular needs;
- to access acceptable, affordable and quality comprehensive healthcare including ART;
- to sexual and reproductive health services, including access to safe abortion without coercion;
- to a broader array of preventive and therapeutic technologies that respond to the needs of all women

Continued on next page

Box 29 (continued)

and girls, regardless of age, HIV status or sexual orientation;
- to access user-friendly and affordable prevention technologies such as female condoms and microbicides with skills building training on negotiation and use;
- to testing after informed consent and protection of confidentiality of their status;
- to choose to disclose their status in circumstances of safety and security without the threat of violence, discrimination and stigma;
- to live their sexuality in safety and with pleasure irrespective of age, HIV status or sexual orientation;
- to choose to be mothers and have children irrespective of their HIV status or sexual orientation;
- to safe and healthy motherhood for all, including the safety and health of their children;
- to choose marriage, form partnerships or divorce, irrespective of age, HIV status or sexual orientation;
- to gender equity in education and lifetime education for all;
- to formal and informal sexual education throughout their lives;
- to information, especially about HIV/AIDS, with an emphasis on women and girl's special vulnerability due to biological differences, gender roles and inequality;
- to employment, equal pay, recognition of all forms of work including sex work and compensation for care and support;
- to economic independence such as to own and inherit property, and to access financial resources;
- to food security, safe water and shelter;
- to freedom of movement and travel irrespective of HIV status;
- to express their religious, cultural and social identities;
- to associate freely and be leaders within religious, social and cultural institutions; and
- to lead and participate in all aspects of politics, governance, decision-making, policy development and programme implementation.

Box 30: Evaluation of poverty- and gender-sensitive HIV/AIDS programmes

- Are women and men accessing VCT? If no, why not?
- How can VCT be made more accessible and affordable to women and men?
- Are people living in poverty able to access HIV/AIDS prevention, care and support services and resources?
- What are the financial barriers in HIV/AIDS prevention, care and support programmes?
- What can be done to ensure that poor people have equal access to HIV/AIDS prevention, care and support services?
- Are women living with HIV/AIDS involved in planning and implementing gender-sensitive HIV/AIDS education, prevention, care and support programmes?
- How can HIV/AIDS prevention, care and support programmes better serve women and girls?
- Are home-based care activities for PLWH shared between male and female family members?
- If women bear most of the burden of family caregiving, what can be done to provide more equitable caregiving responsibilities?
- Is there a programme to provide support for the caregivers (family members, health care practitioners, etc.)? If not, would such a programme be helpful? If yes, how could caregiver support be provided?
- Do young girls and boys access HIV/AIDS education, prevention, care and support services? If not, what can be done to encourage them to do so?
- Are HIV-infected and affected children provided with adequate services? If not, how can such services be improved?
- Are PMTCT services included in MCH and reproductive health programmes? If not, how can these PMTCT be incorporated into health care services?
- Are men involved in PMTCT activities? If not, how can men become involved?
- Are the issues of HIV/AIDS education, prevention and care accessible to older people? If not, how can these services be made available to older people?

Box 31: HIV/AIDS and human rights

- Call for strong and coherent national policies, strategies and regulations to confront gender-driven behaviours. These policies, regulations and legislation should be founded on the principles outlined in the Convention on the Elimination of All Forms of Discrimination (CEDAW).
- Develop effective laws and policies to prohibit trafficking of young women and children.
- Promote non-discriminatory practices in the workplace including refusal to screen workers for HIV.
- Develop legal reforms and other steps aimed at countering the violation of human rights and protecting those infected with and affected by HIV. Such legal reforms should include the right to confidentiality, and the prohibition of forced HIV testing and disclosure. The UNGASS Declaration of Commitment on HIV/AIDS should be used as the foundational document for this work.
- Develop strategies to make governments accountable for their actions in planning and implementing public health policies and programmes that aid in the prevention, care, treatment (including ARV) and support for people living with HIV/AIDS. The UNGASS Declaration of Commitment on HIV/AIDS should be used as the foundational document for this work.
- Promote strategies that lead to the empowerment of vulnerable, marginalized and disenfranchised people (e.g. women, migrants, ethnic minorities, IDUs, sex workers, youth, people living in poverty).
- Place PLWH at the centre of any health policy, programme or legislation that affects the care, support, treatment and prevention of HIV/AIDS. Human rights principles, treaties, conventions, declarations, resolutions, guidelines and recommendations that place the individual at the centre of policies and legislation should be used as the basis for this endeavour.
- Promote free and active participation of people affected by and infected with HIV in the development of policies, regulations and legislation related to HIV/AIDS. This practice should follow a human rights agenda.
- Develop policies and legislation to address stigma and discrimination as a violation of human rights. Freedom from discrimination is a fundamental human right founded on the principles of natural justice.
- Develop policies and legislation that address the rights of the child, whether they are infected with or affected by HIV. The Convention on the Rights of the Child is an important framework for this development. This convention states that children are entitled to the highest attainable standard of health and to facilities for care, prevention, treatment and rehabilitation.
- Enforce the government's obligation to protect people's human rights to: safe and effective health care (including blood safety), information, education, employment and social welfare.
- Reduce people's vulnerability to HIV infection by ensuring humane care, treatment (including ARV) and support for those affected and infected by HIV/AIDS.
- Encourage research into "best practices" at the national and local levels to promote effective, gender-sensitive and culturally appropriate policies, programmes and services for those affected by and infected with HIV. Reports of these practices should be widely disseminated within countries (and internationally) to help promote more responsive care, support, treatment and prevention strategies related to HIV/AIDS.

Box 32: Mainstreaming gender equality and women's human rights: gender in one national AIDS action framework

The following reference points should be considered in either formulating or reviewing a national framework:
- Does the framework fully reflect national and international commitments to increasing gender equality and stopping the spread of HIV?
- Does the framework reinforce existing laws that are in place to advance gender equality and eliminate discrimination (e.g., inheritance, property, employment, etc.)?
- Is the framework based on a gender analysis of the epidemic, reflecting who is getting infected or impacted, and why?
- Does it acknowledge gender disparities in access to prevention, treatment, care, and support, and does it map strategies to address them?
- Does it recognize that protecting women's rights and adjusting power imbalances is fundamental to effective HIV strategies and actions?
- Does it offer particular strategies to reach women, involve men and address gender dynamics present in all areas covered in the framework?
- Does it move beyond a focus on individual behaviour to underscore that gender dynamics, as a social and cultural construct, can often make women more vulnerable to HIV?
- Are there provisions for different groups, including those that may be more vulnerable to HIV due to gender, age, race, economic standing or other factors?
- Does the framework support equality in representation by key stakeholders, at various levels of the response to HIV and AIDS, including the senior decision-making level?
- Were key stakeholders, particularly those from networks of women living with HIV, national ministries tasked with addressing gender equality and women's rights, and groups working on women's rights and gender equality involved in planning, formulating, implementing and monitoring the framework?
- Are there obstacles that hinder women's participation? What steps can be taken to ensure their regular involvement in reviews and monitoring of the framework?
- Does the framework support the inclusion of gender expertise within the national HIV/AIDS coordinating and operational bodies, and HIV expertise within the national mechanism(s) for women and gender equality? Does the framework ensure the involvement of gender equality advocates in the development of monitoring and evaluation strategies?
- Are existing statistical, research and data gathering mechanisms gender-sensitive and do they incorporate evidence and data provided by women's groups, gender advocates and community-based researchers?

Source: United Nations Development Fund for Women 2008.

Box 33. Examples of gender-sensitive HIV/AIDS indicators, with targets and information sources

Gender-sensitive indicators by type	Targets	Information sources
Input indicators (the people, training, equipment and resources needed to achieve outputs): • Amount of HIV/AIDS budget targeting gender-sensitive measures • Sectoral ministries that have incorporated gender-sensitive issues in annual plans • Number of gender-HIV/AIDS trainings for government staff and peer educators • Percent of line ministry staff by sex who are active in HIV/AIDS programmes	• UNGASS Article 61: By 2005, ensure development and accelerated implementation of national strategies for women's empowerment. • By 2004, at least 500 line ministry staff trained	• Annual plans of sectoral ministries • Monitoring, disbursement, or supervision reports
Output indicators (activities and services delivered to achieve outcomes): • Participation of women's organisations in HIV/AIDS policy development, implementation and monitoring • Number of programmes/ organizations providing skills to women and men • Number of gender-sensitive HIV/AIDS prevention programmes integrated into school curricula • Number of stigma reduction activities, and percent of males and females enrolled	• By 2005 increase by 20% the number of organizations providing skills to young women • By end of 2004, increase to x the number of NGOs and CBOs preparing and implementing community and civil society initiatives on gender issues	• Mid-term and supervision reports. • Special studies.
Impact indicators (overall measurable HIV/AIDS impacts, e.g., reduced transmission and prevalence): • Prevalence among 15-24 year old males and females, including pregnant women • Rate of mother-to-child transmission • Life expectancy by sex • Number of girls and boys orphaned by HIV/AIDS	• MDG 6: Have halted by 2015 and begun to reverse the spread of HIV/AIDS • UNGASS Articles 37: By 2003, […] address gender-based dimensions of the epidemic	• Mid-term and supervision reports • Special studies • National statistical reports, UNAIDS, UNICEF, WHO
Outcome indicators (e.g., changes in behaviour or skills needed to achieve outcomes): • Number of women and men who know at least two methods of protection against HIV/AIDS • Number of women who report using a condom with a regular partner during the last 12 months • Proportion of sex workers (male and female) who report condom use with last client	• UNGASS Article 53: By 2005, ensure that at least 90% of men and women aged 15-24 have access to information, education and communication (IEC) • Increase from x% to y% the proportion of sex workers reporting using condoms	• Mid-term and completion evaluation reports • Household and special surveys, such as Behavioral Surveillance Surveys

Source: Joint United Nations Programme on HIV/AIDS Inter-Agency Task Team on Gender and HIV/AIDS, undated.

Resources

Detailed clinical information on prevention, VCT, ART and home-based care can be found in WHO's clinical training manuals on HIV/AIDS and ART for doctors, nurses and allied health workers at the district or intermediate level[0](www.wpro.who.int/health_topics/hiv_infections/publications.htm).

A range of technical resources can be found on the websites of the Joint United Nations Programme on HIV/AIDS (www.unaids.org), WHO Headquarters (www.who.int/hiv/en/) and the WHO Regional Office for the Western Pacific (www.wpro.who.int/health_topics/hiv_infections/).

Some specific technical resources are listed below:

Voluntary testing and counselling:

WHO and the Joint United Nations Programme on HIV/AIDS. *Guidance on provider-initiated HIV testing counselling in health facilities* (http://whqlibdoc.who.int/publications/2007/9789241595568_eng.pdf).

WHO and the Joint United Nations Programme on HIV/AIDS. *Scaling-up HIV testing and counselling services: a toolkit for programme managers* (www.who.int/entity/hiv/pub/vct/counsellingtestingtoolkit.pdf).

Prevention of mother-to-child transmission:

WHO has developed a tool kit to facilitate the integration and delivery of testing and counselling for the prevention of mother-to-child transmission of HIV. It is available at: www.womenchildrenhiv.org/wchiv?page=vc-10-00.

Health system strengthening

WHO has developed a number of guidelines with the aim of strengthening health services to fight HIV/AIDS. One such publication, *Antiretroviral therapy for HIV infection in adults and adolescents: recommendations for a public health approach*, 2006 revision (www.who.int/entity/hiv/pub/guidelines/artadultguidelines.pdf), outlines recommendations for countries to take a public health approach to treatment for HIV.

WHO recommends that national plans to scale up ART should include training for health care professionals on the Integrated Management of Adult Illness. These guidelines can be accessed at: www.who.int/hiv/pub/imai/en/extending_essential_care.pdf.

Poverty, gender and HIV/AIDS:

Eldis (www.eldis.org) provides a searchable database of development resources with a section on HIV/AIDS, including focus areas dedicated to the relationship between poverty and gender and HIV.

BRIDGE (www.bridge.ids.ac.uk), which supports research on gender and development, has produced a number of useful publications that summarize available evidence on gender and HIV, including a recent publication on women living with HIV/AIDS.

The United Nations Development Fund for Women, or UNIFEM, in collaboration with UNAIDS, has developed the **UNIFEM Gender and HIV/AIDS Portal** [www.genderandaids.org] to provide up-to-date information on the gender dimensions of the HIV/AIDS epidemic. The site aims to promote understanding, knowledge sharing, and action on HIV/AIDS as a gender and human rights issue. It contains various resources on the gender dimensions of the HIV/AIDS epidemic, including research studies, training materials, multi-media advocacy tools, speeches and presentations, press releases and current news, best practices and personal stories, campaign actions and opinion pieces by leading commentators.

The **World Bank** supports a number of HIV/AIDS-related projects around the world. Information on these projects, as well as technical guidelines and advocacy reports can be found at: http://web.worldbank.org/WBSITE/EXTERNAL/TOPICS/EXTHEALTHNUTRITIONANDPOPULATION/EXTHIVAIDS/0,,menuPK:376477~pagePK:149018~piPK:149093~theSitePK:376471,00.html

The United Nations Development Fund for Women, or UNIFEM, in collaboration with UNAIDS, has developed the **UNIFEM Gender and HIV/AIDS Portal** [www.genderandaids.org] to provide up-to-date information on the gender dimensions of the HIV/AIDS epidemic. The site aims to promote understanding, knowledge sharing, and action on HIV/AIDS as a gender and human rights issue. It contains various resources on the gender dimensions of the HIV/AIDS epidemic, including research studies, training materials, multi-media advocacy tools, speeches and presentations, press releases and current news, best practices and personal stories, campaign actions and opinion pieces by leading commentators.

The **World Bank** also supports research into inequalities in access to HIV/AIDS prevention, treatment and care and the impact of HIV/AIDS, among other topics. See, for example, the Poverty and Health web page (http://web.worldbank.org/WBSITE/EXTERNAL/TOPICS/EXTHEALTHNUTRITIONANDPOPULATION/EXTPAH/0,,menuPK:400482~pagePK:149018~piPK:149093~theSitePK:400476,00.html).

The **World Health Organization Department for Gender and Women's Health** has a number of resources on gender and HIV/AIDS (http://www.who.int/gender/hiv_aids/en/), including fact sheets on gender and HIV and policy documents on equitable access to ART.

Human rights and HIV/AIDS:

The **World Health Organization** maintains a number of resources on health and human rights, including those specific to gender and HIV/AIDS (www.who.int/topics/human_rights/en/).

The **Office of the United Nations High Commissioner on Human Rights** has considered international human rights treaties with regards to HIV/AIDS (www.ohchr.org/english/issues/hiv/index.htm). The Commission on Human Rights has appointed a Special Rapporteur on the right to health (www.ohchr.org/english/issues/health/right/).

Impact of HIV/AIDS:

Numerous organizations are concerned with the impact of HIV/AIDS on children and youth. The **UNICEF** website (www.unicef.org) has a section dedicated to HIV/AIDS and children. The **International Labour Organization** recently published *HIV/AIDS and work: global estimates, impact* *on children and youth, and response* (www.ilo.org/public/english/protection/trav/aids/publ/global_est06/global_estimates_report06.pdf).

Women and girls living with HIV/AIDS: overview and annotated bibliography, published by BRIDGE, considers the specific challenges faced by HIV-infected women and girls (www.siyanda.org/search/summary.cfm?nn=2760&ST=SS&Keywords=2007&SUBJECT=0&Donor=&StartRow=1&Ref=Sim).

REFERENCES

ActionAid. *Evaluating stepping stones: a review of existing evaluations and ideas for future M and E work.* Johannesburg, ActionAid International, 2006.

ActionAid. *Time to Act: HIV/AIDS in Asia.* Bangkok, ActionAid, 2005.

Adeyi O. et al. *AIDS, poverty reduction and debt relief. A toolkit for mainstreaming HIV/AIDS programmes into development instruments.* Geneva, UNAIDS, 2001.

Aggleton P. et al. *Bisexualities and AIDS: international perspectives.* London, Taylor & Francis, 1996.

Aggleton P., Warwick I. Community responses to AIDS. In: Joint United Nations Programme on HIV/AIDS. *Sex and youth: contextual factors affecting risk for HIV/AIDS.* Geneva, UNAIDS, 1999(library.unesco-iicba.org/English/HIV_AIDS/cdrom%20materials/PDFfiles/99sandy1.pdf, accessed 26 February 2007).

Agha S. An evaluation of adolescent sexual health programmes in Cameroon, Botswana, South Africa, and Guinea. *PSI Research Division Working Paper 29.* Washington D.C., Population Services International, 2000.

Alford S. et al. *Science and success in developing countries: holistic programmes that work to prevent teen pregnancy, HIV and sexually transmitted infections.* Washington D.C., Advocates for Youth, 2005.

Antiretroviral therapy/3 by 5 Initiative. Manila, World Health Organization Regional Office for the Western Pacific, 2005 (http://www.wpro.who.int/health_topics/antiretroviral_therapy/general_info.htm, accessed 23 February 2007).

Ashford L. *Social marketing for adolescent sexual health. Results of operations research projects in Botswana, Cameroon, Guinea, and South Africa.* Washington D.C., Population Reference Bureau and Population Services International, 2000.

Asian Development Bank. *Indigenous Peoples/Ethnic Minorities and Poverty Reduction: Pacific Region.* Manila, ADB, 2002a.

Asian Development Bank. *Indigenous Peoples/Ethnic Minorities and Poverty Reduction: Viet Nam.* Manila, ADB, 2002b.

Asian Development Bank. *Indigenous Peoples/Ethnic Minorities and Poverty Reduction: Cambodia.* Manila, ADB, 2002c.

Asian Development Bank. *Indigenous Peoples/Ethnic Minorities and Poverty Reduction: The Philippines.* Manila, ADB, 2002d.

Asian Development Bank. Health and education needs of the ethnic minorities in the Greater Mekong Subregion. Manila, ADB, 2001.

Australian Agency for International Development and United Nations Development Programme. *Impact of HIV/AIDS on household vulnerability and poverty in Viet Nam.* Hanoi, United Nations Development Programme Viet Nam, 2005 (VIE/98/006).

Barker G. *Listening to Boys: Some Reflections on Adolescent Boys and Gender Equity.* Paper presented at the AWID Conference Panel "Male Involvement in Sexual and Reproductive Health: Hindrance or Help to Gender Equity?" Washington, D.C., 12 November 1999.

Beegle K., De Weerdt J., Dercon S. Adult mortality and consumption growth in the age of HIV/AIDS. *World Bank Policy Research Working Paper 4082*. Washington D.C., World Bank, 2006.

Bloom D., River Path Associates, Sevilla J. *Health, wealth, AIDS and poverty*. Manila and Geneva, UNAIDS and Asian Development Bank, 2002 (www2.unescobkk.org/hivaids/FullTextDB/aspUploadFiles/HWAP.pdf, accessed 26 February 2007).

Bloom D., River Path Associates, Sevilla J. *Health, wealth, AIDS and poverty – the case of Cambodia*. Manila and Geneva, UNAIDS and Asian Development Bank, 2001 (http://www.adb.org/Documents/Reports/HW_Cambodia/HWCAM.pdf, accessed 26 February 2007).

Bonnel R. *Background paper: economic analysis of HIV/AIDS*. Washington D.C., World Bank AIDS Campaign Team for Africa, 2000.

Braveman P., Gruskin S. Poverty, equity, human rights and health. *Bulletin of the World Health Organization*, 2003a, 81(7):539–545.

Braveman P., Gruskin S. Theory and methods: defining equity in health. *Journal of Epidemiology and Community Health*, 2003b, 57:254–258.

BRIDGE. *Development and gender brief 10: Culture*. Brighton, Institute of Development Studies, 2002 (http://www.bridge.ids.ac.uk/dgb10.html, accessed 23 February 2007).

Campbell C., Macphail C. Peer education, gender and the development of critical consciousness: participatory HIV prevention by South African youth. *Social Science and Medicine,* 2002, 55:331–345.

Cash K., Anasuchatkul B. *Experimental educational interventions for AIDS prevention among northern Thai single migratory female factory workers*. Washington, D.C., International Center for Research on Women. Women and AIDS Programme Research Report Series, No. 9. 1995.

Centre for HIV/AIDS Networking. *Risking death to stay alive*. Durban, Centre for HIV/AIDS Networking, University of KwaZulu-Natal, 2005 (http://www.hivan.org.za/arttemp.asp?id=1489, accessed 23 February 2007).

Chalker J. *et al*. STD management by private pharmacies in Hanoi: practice and knowledge of drug sellers. *Sexually Transmitted Infection*, 2000, 76:299–302.

Chesney M.A., Smith A.W. Critical delays in HIV testing and care. *American Behavioral Scientist*, 1999, 42:1162–1174.

David Lowe Consulting-Asia. *Perceptions of the Cambodian 100% Condom Use Program: documenting the experience of sex workers*. A report to the POLICY project. March 2003.

DeCarlo P. Protecting mothers and children. *Harvard AIDS Review*, 2000, Spring-Summer: 8–11.

De Cock, K.M. *et al*. Prevention of mother-to-child HIV transmission in resource-poor countries. *Journal of American Medical Association,* 2002, 283(9):1175–1182.

Desbarats J. HIV/AIDS and poverty: the impact of HIV/AIDS in the ESCAP Region. In: Fifth Asian and Pacific Population Conference: Selected Papers. *Asian Population Studies Series No. 158*. New York, Economic and Social Commission for Asia and the Pacific, 2003 (http://www.unescap.org/esid/psis/population/popseries/apss158/index.asp, accessed 23 February 2007).

Dolan K. et al. *Review of injection drug users and HIV infection in prisons in developing and transitional countries*. Sydney, Central and Eastern Europe Harm Reduction Network, August 2004 (www.ceehrn.org/EasyCEE/sys/files/IDUand%20 HIV%20in%20prisons,%20refgr.pdf, accessed 26 February 2007).

Duvvury N., Knoess J. *Gender based violence and HIV/AIDS in Cambodia: links, opportunities and potential responses*. Washington D.C., International Center for Research on Women and GTZ BACKUP Initiative, 2005 (http://www.gtz.de/ dokumente/en-01526-kh-report-2005-08.pdf, accessed 23 February 2007).

Dwyer G. PNG's quiet killer: the rapid spread of HIV/AIDS has prompted urgent action to set up pilot clinics. Manila, *ADB Review*, March-April 2004 (http://www.adb.org/Documents/Periodicals/ADB_Review/2004/vol36_2/health.asp, accessed 2 February 2007).

Engender Health. Men as Partners. New York, Engender Health, 2006 (http://www.engenderhealth.org/ia/wwm/index.htm accessed 23 February 2007).

Esplen E. Women and girls living with HIV/AIDS: overview and annotated bibliography. *BRIDGE (development - gender) Bibliography No. 18.* Brighton, Institute of Development Studies, International Community of Women Living with HIV/ AIDS, 2007.

Family Health International. *Current issues in HIV counselling and testing in South and Southeast Asia.* Report of a workshop in Mumbai, India. Arlington, Population Council and Family Health International, 2000.

Family Health International. *HIV/AIDS care and treatment: a clinical course for people caring for persons living with HIV/AIDS. Facilitator's guide.* Arlington, Family Health International, 2004 (http://www.fhi.org/NR/rdonlyres/ ehdborxsewuavrpjv6iv562fbcwjghnubdjz76tigcrg2xvkscu7uz7xxcg3emjl3aggj3eg2yc6mo/FHICompleteMaryLyn2.pdf, accessed 22 February 2007).

Ford N., Koetsawang S. The sociocultural context of the transmission of HIV in Thailand. *Social Science and Medicine*, 199 33 (4):405–414.

Global Fund to Fight AIDS, Tuberculosis and Malaria. Funded programmes. Geneva, Global Fund, 2006 (http://www. theglobalfund.org/programs/search.aspx?lang=en, accessed 23 February 2007).

Goodman L.A. et al. Male violence against women: current research and future directions. *American Psychologist*, 1993, 48:1054–1058.

Gordon P., Sleightholme C. *Review of 'best practice' for intervention in sexual health.* New Delhi, British Overseas Development Administration Health and Population Office (undated).

Government of the Lao People's Democratic Republic and the United Nations. *Millennium Development Goals Progress Repo Lao PDR*. Vientiane, Government of the Lao People's Democratic Republic and the United Nations, 2004.

Government of Mongolia. *Economic growth support and poverty reduction strategy*. Ulaanbaatar, Government of Mongolia, 2003.

Government of Mongolia and United Nations Development Programme. *Human development report Mongolia 2003: urban-rural disparities in Mongolia*. Ulaanbaatar, United Nations Development Programme, 2003.

Government of Papua New Guinea and United Nations in Papua New Guinea. *Millennium Development Goals progress repo 2004.* Port Moresby, Government of Papua New Guinea and United Nations in Papua New Guinea, 2004.

Government of Papua New Guinea. *The 2007 estimation report on the HIV epidemic in Papua New Guinea*. Port Moresby,

Government of Papua New Guinea, 2007.

Gwatkin D. *Who would gain most from efforts to reach the Millennium Development Goals for health? An inquiry into the possibility of progress that fails to reach the poor*. Health, Nutrition and Population Discussion Paper. Washington, D.C., World Bank, 2002.

Gwatkin D. *et al. Socioeconomic differences in health, nutrition, and population in Cambodia*. Washington, D.C.: World Bank, 2007a.

Gwatkin D. *et al. Socioeconomic differences in health, nutrition, and population in Philippines*. Washington, D.C.: World Bank, 2007b.

Gwatkin D. *et al. Socioeconomic differences in health, nutrition, and population in Vietnam*. Washington, D.C.: World Bank, 2007c.

International Coalition on AIDS and Development. HIV/AIDS and food security. Ottawa, International Coalition on AIDS and Development, 2001 (http://www.icadcisd.com/content/pub_printerfriendly.cfm?PubID=9&CAT=9&lang=e, accessed 19 June 2007).

Hardon A. *et al*. From access to adherence: the challenges of antiretroviral treatment: studies from Botswana, Tanzania and Uganda 2006. Geneva, World Health Organization, 2006 (http://www.eldis.org/cf/rdr/rdr.cfm?doc=DOC22158, accessed 26 February 2007).

He N. *et al*. Sexual behaviour among employed male rural migrants in Shanghai, China. *AIDS Education and Prevention*, 2006, 18(2):176–186.

Health Action Information Network. *2005 Philippine HIV and AIDS country profile*. Health Action Information Network, Philippine National AIDS Council, UNAIDS Philippines, 2005.

HelpAge International. *State of the world's older people*. London, HelpAge International 2002.

Huang M. *HIV/AIDS among fishers: vulnerability of their partners*. Global Symposium on Women in Fisheries, World Fish Centre, 2002.

Human Development Network. *Philippines Human Development Report 2005*. Manila, Human Development Network, 2005.

Human Rights Watch. India: AIDS fuelled by abuses against children, children affected by HIV/AIDS face lethal discrimination and exploitation. New York, Human Rights Watch, 2006 (http://hrw.org/english/docs/2004/07/29/india9156.htm, accessed 23 February 2007).

Human Rights Watch. Human Rights Watch Prison Project. New York, Human Rights Watch, n.d. (http://www.hrw.org/advocacy/prisons/hiv-aids.htm, accessed 23 February 2007).

Hunter S., Williamson J. *Children on the brink: strategies to support children isolated by HIV/AIDS*. Washington, D.C., United States Agency for International Development, 1997.

Id21. HIV/AIDS, poverty and schooling: an AIDS epidemic or a poverty epidemic? Brighton, Institute of Development Studies, 2002a (http://www.id21.org/society/S5cbg1g1.html, accessed 26 February 2007).

Id21. No quick fix: tackling the AIDS epidemic through combating poverty. Brighton, Institute of Development Studies, 2002b (http://www.id21.org/society/S5bei1g1.html, accessed 26 February 2007).

Id21. *Meeting their needs? Discussing young people's sexual health*. Brighton, Institute of Development Studies, 2002c (ttp://www.id21.org/health/E5iw1g1.html, accessed 26 February 2007).

Id21. Place matters: the challenges of survival in remote rural areas. Brighton, Institute of Development Studies, 2002d (http://www.id21.org/society/s5bkb1g1.html, accessed 26 February 2007).

International Labour Organization and World Health Organization. *Draft joint ILO/WHO guidelines on health services and HIV/AIDS*. Geneva, ILO and WHO, 2005.

The International Community of Women Living with HIV/AIDS. *HIV Positive Women, Poverty, and Gender Inequality*. ICW Vision Paper 3. London, The International Community of Women Living with HIV/AIDS, 2004 (http://www.icw.org/tiki-download_file.php?fileId=62, accessed 23 February 2007).

Joint United Nations Programme on HIV/AIDS. *The UNAIDS guide to the United Nations human rights machinery*. Geneva, UNAIDS, 1997a.

Joint United Nations Programme on HIV/AIDS. *Report from a consultation on the socioeconomic impact of HIV/AIDS on households*. Geneva, UNAIDS, 1997b.

Joint United Nations Programme on HIV/AIDS. *Women and AIDS: UNAIDS point of view* (UNAIDS Best Practice Collection). Geneva, UNAIDS, 1997c.

Joint United Nations Programme on HIV/AIDS. *Prisons and AIDS* (UNAIDS Best Practice Collection). Geneva, UNAIDS, 1997d.

Joint United Nations Programme on HIV/AIDS. *Community mobilization and AIDS* (UNAIDS Best Practice Collection). Geneva, UNAIDS, 1997e.

Joint United Nations Programme on HIV/AIDS. *Refugees and AIDS* (UNAIDS Best Practice Collection). Geneva, UNAIDS, 1997f.

Joint United Nations Programme on HIV/AIDS. *Expanding the global response to HIV/AIDS through focused action: Reducing risk and vulnerability: definitions, rationale and pathways*. Geneva, UNAIDS, 1998a.

Joint United Nations Programme on HIV/AIDS. *Putting HIV/AIDS on the business agenda* (UNAIDS Best Practice Collection). Geneva, UNAIDS, 1998b.

Joint United Nations Programme on HIV/AIDS. *Cost-effectiveness analysis and HIV/AIDS* (UNAIDS Best Practice Collection). Geneva, UNAIDS, 1998c.

Joint United Nations Programme on HIV/AIDS. *Gender and HIV/AIDS* (UNAIDS Best Practice Collection). Geneva, UNAIDS, 1998d.

Joint United Nations Programme on HIV/AIDS. *Facing the challenges of HIV/AIDS/STDs: a gender-based response*. KIT, SAFAIDS, UNAIDS, 1998e.

Joint United Nations Programme on HIV/AIDS. *Guide to the strategic planning process for a national response to HIV/AIDS*. Geneva, UNAIDS, 1998f.

Joint United Nations Programme on HIV/AIDS. *AIDS and the military* (UNAIDS Best Practice Collection). Geneva, UNAIDS, 1998g.

Joint United Nations Programme on HIV/AIDS. *A measure of success in Uganda: the value of monitoring both HIV prevalence and sexual behaviour.* Geneva, UNAIDS, 1998h.

Joint United Nations Programme on HIV/AIDS. *Partners in prevention: international case studies of effective health promotion practice in HIV/AIDS.* Geneva, UNAIDS, 1998i.

Joint United Nations Programme on HIV/AIDS. *Guide to the strategic planning process for a national response to HIV/AIDS: Strategic plan formulation.* Geneva, UNAIDS, 1999a.

Joint United Nations Programme on HIV/AIDS. *Handbook for legislators on HIV/AIDS, law and human rights.* Geneva, UNAIDS, 1999b.

Joint United Nations Programme on HIV/AIDS. *Communications framework for HIV/AIDS: A new direction.* A UNAIDS/Penn State Project. Geneva, UNAIDS, 1999c.

Joint United Nations Programme on HIV/AIDS. *School health education to prevent AIDS and STD. A resource package for curriculum planners.* Geneva, UNAIDS, 1999d.

Joint United Nations Programme on HIV/AIDS. *Knowledge is power: voluntary HIV counselling and testing in Uganda.* Geneva, UNAIDS, 1999e.

Joint United Nations Programme on HIV/AIDS. *Peer education and HIV/AIDS: concepts, uses and challenges.* Geneva, UNAIDS, 1999f.

Joint United Nations Programme on HIV/AIDS. *Evaluation of a national AIDS programme: a methods package.* Geneva, UNAIDS, 1999g.

Joint United Nations Programme on HIV/AIDS. *Vulnerability of girl children and HIV/AIDS: the Thai approach.* Geneva, UNAIDS, 1999h.

Joint United Nations Programme on HIV/AIDS. *Sex and youth: contextual factors affecting risk for HIV/AIDS.* Geneva, UNAIDS, 1999i.

Joint United Nations Programme on HIV/AIDS. *Reducing girl's vulnerability to HIV/AIDS: the Thai approach.* UNAIDS Case Study. Geneva, UNAIDS, 1999j.

Joint United Nations Programme on HIV/AIDS. *HIV/AIDS: emerging issues and challenges for women, young people and infants.* Geneva, UNAIDS, 1999k.

Joint United Nations Programme on HIV/AIDS. *Gender and AIDS: taking stock of research and programmes.* Geneva, UNAIDS, 1999m.

Joint United Nations Programme on HIV/AIDS. *A review of household and community responses to HIV/AIDS epidemic in the rural areas of sub-Saharan Africa.* Geneva, UNAIDS, 1999n.

Joint United Nations Programme on HIV/AIDS. *Sexual behavioural change for HIV: Where have the theories taken us?* Geneva, UNAIDS, 1999o.

Joint United Nations Programme on HIV/AIDS. *Launching and promoting the female condom in Eastern and Southern Africa* Geneva, UNAIDS, 1999p.

Joint United Nations Programme on HIV/AIDS. *Trends in HIV incidence and prevalence: natural course of the epidemic or results of behavioural change?* Geneva, UNAIDS, 1999q.

Joint United Nations Programme on HIV/AIDS. *Report on the global HIV/AIDS epidemic (June 2000).* Geneva, UNAIDS, 2000a.

Joint United Nations Programme on HIV/AIDS. *Guide to the strategic planning process for a national response to HIV/AIDS: Resource mobilization.* Geneva, UNAIDS, 2000b.

Joint United Nations Programme on HIV/AIDS. *A human rights approach to AIDS prevention at work: the southern African development community's code on HIV/AIDS and employment.* Geneva, UNAIDS, 2000c.

Joint United Nations Programme on HIV/AIDS. *Putting knowledge to work: technical resource networks for effective response to HIV/AIDS.* Geneva, UNAIDS, 2000d.

Joint United Nations Programme on HIV/AIDS. *Guidelines for studies on the social and economic impact of HIV/AIDS.* Geneva, UNAIDS, 2000e.

Joint United Nations Programme on HIV/AIDS. *The business response to HIV/AIDS: impact and lessons learned.* Geneva, UNAIDS, 2000f.

Joint United Nations Programme on HIV/AIDS. *Economics and AIDS in Africa: getting priorities right (ADF).* Geneva, UNAIDS, 2000g.

Joint United Nations Programme on HIV/AIDS. *Economics in HIV/AIDS planning: getting priorities right.* Geneva, UNAIDS, Geneva 2000h.

Joint United Nations Programme on HIV/AIDS. *Costing guidelines for HIV prevention strategies.* Geneva, UNAIDS, 2000i.

Joint United Nations Programme on HIV/AIDS. *Tools for evaluating HIV voluntary counselling and testing.* Geneva, UNAIDS, 2000j.

Joint United Nations Programme on HIV/AIDS. *National AIDS programme: a guide to monitoring and evaluation.* Geneva, UNAIDS, 2000k.

Joint United Nations Programme on HIV/AIDS. *Men make a difference: objectives and ideas for action.* Geneva, UNAIDS, 2000m.

Joint United Nations Programme on HIV/AIDS. *Men and AIDS, a gendered approach.* Geneva, UNAIDS, 2000n.

Joint United Nations Programme on HIV/AIDS. *AIDS and men who have sex with men: technical update.* Geneva, UNAIDS, 2000o.

Joint United Nations Programme on HIV/AIDS. *Protocol for the identification of discrimination against people with HIV* Geneva, UNAIDS, 2000p.

Joint United Nations Programme on HIV/AIDS. *From principle to practice: greater involvement of people living with or affected by HIV/AIDS.* Geneva, UNAIDS, 2000q.

Joint United Nations Programme on HIV/AIDS. *Migrant populations and HIV/AIDS: the development and implementation of programmes: theory, methodology and practices.* Geneva, UNAIDS, 2000r.

Joint United Nations Programme on HIV/AIDS. *Discussion paper on models for VCT for MTCT interventions in Eastern Europe.* Geneva, UNAIDS, 2000s.

Joint United Nations Programme on HIV/AIDS. *Innovative approaches to HIV prevention: selected case studies.* Geneva, UNAIDS, 2000t.

Joint United Nations Programme on HIV/AIDS. *The 100% condom programme in Thailand.* Geneva, UNAIDS, 2000u.

Joint United Nations Programme on HIV/AIDS. *The female condom: a guide for planning and programming.* Geneva, UNAIDS, 2000v.

Joint United Nations Programme on HIV/AIDS. *HIV and AIDS-related stigmatization, discrimination and denial.* Geneva, UNAIDS, 2000w.

Joint United Nations Programme on HIV/AIDS. *AIDS epidemic update 2001.* Geneva, UNAIDS, 2001.

Joint United Nations Programme on HIV/AIDS. *AIDS, poverty reduction and debt relief: A toolkit for mainstreaming HIV/AIDS programmes into development instruments.* Geneva, UNAIDS, 2001a.

Joint United Nations Programme on HIV/AIDS. *Young people and AIDS.* Geneva, UNAIDS, 2001b.

Joint United Nations Programme on HIV/AIDS. *Resource packet on gender and AIDS.* Geneva, UNAIDS, 2001c.

Joint United Nations Programme on HIV/AIDS. *Population mobility and AIDS: technical update.* Geneva, UNAIDS, 2001d.

Joint United Nations Programme on HIV/AIDS. *Report on the global HIV/AIDS epidemic: The Barcelona Report, UNAIDS: XIV International Conference on AIDS, Barcelona.* Geneva, UNAIDS, 2002a.

Joint United Nations Programme on HIV/AIDS. New UNAIDS report warns AIDS epidemic still in early phase and not levelling off in worst affected countries. Geneva, UNAIDS, 2002b (http://www.aegis.com/news/unaids/2002/UN020701.html, accessed 26 February 2007).

Joint United Nations Programme on HIV/AIDS. *Handbook on access to HIV/AIDS-related treatment: a collection of information, tools and other resources for NGOs, CBOs and PLWHA groups.* Geneva and Brighton, UNAIDS, World Health Organization and International HIV/AIDS Alliance, 2003.

Joint United Nations Programme on HIV/AIDS. *AIDS epidemic update 2004.* Geneva. UNAIDS, 2004a.

Joint United Nations Programme on HIV/AIDS. *Women and AIDS fact sheet.* Geneva, UNAIDS, 2004b.

Joint United Nations Programme on HIV/AIDS. *Men who have sex with men, HIV prevention and care.* Report of a UNAIDS stakeholder consultation. Geneva, 10-11 November 2005. Geneva, UNAIDS, 2005.

Joint United Nations Programme on HIV/AIDS. *AIDS epidemic update: special report on HIV/AIDS: December 2006.* Geneva, UNAIDS and WHO, 2006a.

Joint United Nations Programme on HIV/AIDS. *UNAIDS statement on the political declaration on HIV/AIDS.* Geneva, UNAIDS, 2006b (http://data.unaids.org/pub/PressStatement/2006/20060620_PS_HLM_en.pdf, accessed 1 December 2006).

Joint United Nations Programme on HIV/AIDS. *UNAIDS policy brief: HIV and sex between men*. Geneva, UNAIDS, 2006c (http://data.unaids.org/pub/BriefingNote/2006/20060801_Policy_Brief_MSM_en.pdf, accessed 7 December 2006).

Joint United Nations Programme on HIV/AIDS. *Setting national targets for moving towards universal access. Operational Guidance*. Geneva, UNAIDS, 2006d.

Joint United Nations Programme on HIV/AIDS. *2006 report on the global AIDS epidemic: a UNAIDS 10th anniversary special edition*. Geneva, UNAIDS, 2006e.

Joint United Nations Programme on HIV/AIDS. *Scaling up access to HIV prevention, treatment, care and support: the next steps*. Geneva, UNAIDS, 2006f.

Joint United Nations Programme on HIV/AIDS. *Epidemiological fact sheet on HIV/AIDS and sexually transmitted infections: Cambodia*. European Union, UNAIDS, United Nations Children's Fund, World Health Organization, 2006g.

Joint United Nations Programme on HIV/AIDS. *Epidemiological fact sheet on HIV/AIDS and sexually transmitted infections: China*. European Union, UNAIDS, United Nations Children's Fund, World Health Organization, 2006h.

Joint United Nations Programme on HIV/AIDS. *Epidemiological fact sheet on HIV/AIDS and sexually transmitted infections: Malaysia*. European Union, UNAIDS, United Nations Children's Fund, World Health Organization, 2006i.

Joint United Nations Programme on HIV/AIDS. *Epidemiological fact sheet on HIV/AIDS and sexually transmitted infections: Philippines*. European Union, UNAIDS, United Nations Children's Fund, World Health Organization, 2006j.

Joint United Nations Programme on HIV/AIDS. *Epidemiological fact sheet on HIV/AIDS and sexually transmitted infections: Papua New Guinea*. European Union, UNAIDS, United Nations Children's Fund, World Health Organization, 2006k.

Joint United Nations Programme on HIV/AIDS. *Epidemiological fact sheet on HIV/AIDS and sexually transmitted infections: Viet Nam*. European Union, UNAIDS, United Nations Children's Fund, World Health Organization, 2006l.

Joint United Nations Programme on HIV/AIDS. Children. Geneva, UNAIDS, 2007a (http://www.unaids.org/en/Issues/Affected_communities/default.asp, accessed 23 February 2007).

Joint United Nations Programme on HIV/AIDS. Counselling and Testing. Geneva, UNAIDS, 2007b (http://www.unaids.org/en/Policies/Testing/default.asp, accessed 23 February 2007).

Joint United Nations Programme on HIV/AIDS. Microbicides. Geneva, UNAIDS, 2007c (http://www.unaids.org/en/Issues/Research/Microbicides.asp, accessed 22 February 2007).

Joint United Nations Programme on HIV/AIDS. Orphans. Geneva, UNAIDS, 2007d (http://www.unaids.org/en/Issues/Affected_communities/orphans.asp, accessed 23 February 2007).

Joint United Nations Programme on HIV/AIDS. Prisons. Geneva, UNAIDS, 2007e (http://www.unaids.org/

en/Issues/Affected_communities/prisons.asp, accessed 23 February 2007).

Joint United Nations Programme on HIV/AIDS. The Three Ones. Geneva, UNAIDS, 2007f (http://www.unaids.org/en/Coordination/Initiatives/three_ones.asp, 23 February 2007).

Joint United Nations Programme on HIV/AIDS. *AIDS epidemic update: 2007*. Geneva, UNAIDS and WHO, 2007g.

Joint United Nations Programme on HIV/AIDS. *2008 report on the global AIDS epidemic, UNAIDS-WHO (2007 data)*. Geneva, UNAIDS and WHO, 2008.

Joint United Nations Programme on HIV/AIDS Inter-Agency Task Team on Gender and HIV/AIDS. Resource Pack: 17 Fact Sheets with concise information on gender-related aspects of AIDS. Undated publication (available at: http://www.genderandaids.org/downloads/events/Fact%20Sheets.pdf, accessed 16 September 2008).

Joint United Nations Programme on HIV/AIDS, United Nations Development Programme and World Bank. *Mainstreaming AIDS in development instruments and processes at the national level: a review of experiences*. Geneva, New York and Washington, UNAIDS, UNDP and World Bank, 2005.

Joint United Nations Programme on HIV/AIDS and World Health Organization. *2004 report on the global HIV/AIDS epidemic: 4th global report*. Geneva, UNAIDS, 2004a.

Joint United Nations Programme on HIV/AIDS and World Health Organization. *Policy statement on HIV testing*. Geneva, UNAIDS and WHO, 2004b (http://www.who.int/entity/hiv/pub/vct/en/hivtestingpolicy04.pdf, accessed 7 December 2006).

Joint United Nations Programme on HIV/AIDS and World Health Organization. *WHO and UNAIDS Secretariat statement on HIV testing and counselling*. Geneva, UNAIDS and WHO, 2006a (http://www.who.int/hiv/toronto2006/WHO-UNAIDSstatement_TC_081406_dh.pdf, accessed 7 December 2006).

Joint United Nations Programme on HIV/AIDS and World Health Organization. *Progress on global access to HIV antiretroviral therapy: a report on "3 by 5" and beyond*. Geneva, WHO, 2006b.

Joint United Nations Programme on HIV/AIDS and World Health Organization. *2006 report on the global HIV/AIDS epidemic: 4th global report*. Geneva, UNAIDS, 2006c.

Jurgens R., Cohen J. *Human Rights and HIV/AIDS: now more than ever. 10 reasons why human rights should occupy the center of the global AIDS struggle*. New York, Law and Health Initiative, Open Society Institute, Public Health Programme, n.d.

Kamali A. *et al.* A community randomised trial to investigate impact of improved STD management and behavioural interventions on HIV incidence in rural Masaka district, Uganda: trial design, methods and baseline findings, *Tropical Medicine and International Health*, 2002, 7:1053–1063.

Kaufman J., Jing J. China and AIDS – The Time to Act is Now. *Science*, 2002, 296:2339–2340.

Knodel J. *Poverty and the impact of AIDS on older persons: evidence from Cambodia and Thailand*. Ann Arbor, University of Michigan, 2005 (http://www.psc.isr.umich.edu/pubs/pdf/rr06-597.pdf, accessed 23 February 2007).

Korean UNAIDS Information Support Centre. *Migration and HIV: vulnerability assessment among foreign migrants in South Korea.* Seoul, Korean UNAIDS Information Support Centre 2004.

Krueger L. *et al.* Poverty and HIV seroposivity: the poor are more likely to be infected. *AIDS*, 1990, 4(8):811–814.

Kumarasamy N. *et al.* Barriers and facilitators to antiretroviral medication adherence among patients with HIV in Chennai, India: a qualitative study. *AIDS Patient Care and STD*, 2005, 19(8):526–537.

Lacey C. *et al.*, Analysis of the sociodemography of gonorrhoea in Leeds. *British Medical Journal,* 1997, 314 (1):715–18.

Lampietti J., Stalker L. *Consumption expenditure and female poverty: a review of the evidence.* Policy Research Report on Gender and Development Working Paper Series No. 11. Washington D.C., World Bank, 2000.

Lao People's Democratic Republic. *National Poverty Eradication Programme.* Vientiane, Lao People's Democratic Republic, 2003.

Lau J.T.F., Tsul H.Y. Discriminatory attitudes towards people living with HIV/AIDS and associated factors: a population based study in the Chinese general population. *Sexually Transmitted Infections*, 2005, 81:113–119.

Lightfoot C., Ryan T. Is poverty an issue in the Pacific? Paper presented at the Asia and Pacific Forum on Poverty: Reforming Policies and Institutions for Poverty Reduction. Manila, Asian Development Bank, 2001 (http://www.adb.org/Poverty/Forum/frame_lightfoot.htm, accessed 23 February 2007).

MacNaughton G. Women's human rights related to health-care services in the context of HIV/AIDS. *Health and Human Rights Working Paper Series No. 5.* Geneva, World Health Organization, 2004.

Maman S. *et al.* HIV and partner violence: implications for HIV voluntary counseling and testing programmes in Dar es Salaam, Tanzania. New York, Population Council, 2001 (http://www.popcouncil.org/pdfs/horizons/vctviolence.pdf, accessed 26 February 2007).

Mane P. *Women to gender: from rhetoric to action in HIV/AIDS prevention, care, support and impact alleviation* Paper presented at the Third International Conference on Biopsychosocial Aspects of HIV Infection. Melbourne, Medical Foundation for AIDS & Sexual Health, 22–25 June 1997.

Masanjala W. The poverty-HIV/AIDS nexus in Africa: a livelihood approach. *Social Science and Medicine*, 2007, 64:1032–1041.

Mateo, Jr. R. *et al. HIV/AIDS in the Philippines.* Manila, Remedios AIDS Foundation, 2004 (http://www.remedios.com.ph/fhtml/hivstat_articles.htm, accessed 23 February 2007).

McCamish M., Storer G., Carl G. Refocusing HIV/AIDS interventions in Thailand. *Culture, Health and Sexuality.* 2000, 2(2):167–82.

McMurry C. *Situation of children, youth and women in the Solomon Islands: 2004 Update.* Honiara, Solomon Islands Government and UNICEF, 2004.

Medical Foundation for AIDS & Sexual Health. *Recommended standards for NHS HIV services.* London, Medical Foundation for AIDS & Sexual Health (MedFASH), 2003 (www.medfash.org.uk/publications/documents/Recommended_standards_for_NHS_HIV_services.pdf, accessed 26 February 2007).

Ministry of Planning, Kingdom of Cambodia. *National Human Development Report Cambodia: Societal Aspects of the HIV/AIDS Epidemic in Cambodia, Progress Report 2001.* Phnom Penh, United Nations Development Programme, 2001.

Monitoring the AIDS Pandemic Network. *The status and trends of HIV/AIDS/STI epidemics in Asia and the Pacific.* Melbourne, Monitoring the AIDS Pandemic Network, 2001 (http://www.thebody.com/unaids/pdfs/asia_trends.pdf, accessed 23 February 2007).

Nath, Madhubala. Women's health and HIV: experiences from a sex workers' project in Calcutta. *Gender and Development,* 2000, 8(1). In: Tallis V. *Gender and HIV/AIDS: overview report.* Brighton, Institute of Development Studies, 2002.

Napravnik S. *et al.* Gender difference in HIV RNA levels: a meta-analysis of published studies. *Journal of Acquired Immune Deficiency Syndrome*, 2002, 31(1):11–19.

Office of the United Nations High Commissioner for Human Rights. *General Comment No. 14. The right to the highest attainable standard of health* (article 12 of the International Convention on Economic, Social and Cultural Rights). Geneva, Office of the United Nations High Commissioner for Human Rights, 2000 (http://www.unhchr.ch/tbs/doc.nsf/(symbol)/E.C.12.2000.4.En?OpenDocument, accessed 23 February 2007).

Organisation for Economic Co-operation and Development and World Health Organization. *DAC guidelines and reference series: poverty and health.* Paris, OECD Development Assistance Committee, 2003.

Orubuloye I.O., Caldwell J.C., Caldwell P. African women's control over their sexuality in an era of AIDS: a study of Nigeria. *Social Science and Medicine*, 1993, 37:859–872.

Panos Institute. *Young Men and HIV - culture, poverty and sexual risk.* Briefing no. 41. London, Panos Institute, 2001.

Passey M. *et al.* Community based study of sexually transmitted diseases in rural women in the highlands of Papua New Guinea: prevalence and risk factors. *Sexually Transmitted Infections*, 1998, 74:120–127.

Paxton S. *et al.* "Oh! This one is infected!": Women, HIV & human rights in the Asia-Pacific Region. Paper presented at the Expert Meeting on HIV/AIDS and Human Rights in Asia-Pacific, Bangkok, 23–24 March 2004 (www.un.or.th/ohchr/issues/hivaids/hivaidsmain.html, accessed 16 February 2007).

Physicians for Human Rights. *Guide to using the Global Fund to Fight AIDS, Tuberculosis and Malaria to support health systems strengthening in Round 6.* Washington D.C, Physicians for Human Rights, 2006 (http://physiciansforhumanrights.org/library/documents/reports/using-the-global-fund.pdf, accessed 26 February 2007).

Population Council. *HIV voluntary counselling and testing among youth ages 14 to 21: results from an exploratory study in Nairobi, Kenya, and Kampala and Masaka, Uganda.* Horizons Programme. Population Council, 2001 (www.popcouncil.org/pdfs/horizons/vctyouthbaseline.pdf, accessed 27 February 2006).

Preble E.A., Piwoz E.G. *Prevention of mother-to-child transmission of HIV in Asia: practical guidance for programmes.* Washington, D.C., The LINKAGES Project, 2002.

Price N. The performance of social marketing in reaching the poor and vulnerable in AIDS control programmes. *Health and Policy Planning*, 2001, 16(3):231–239.

Remedios AIDS Foundation. Populations at Risk. Manila, Remedios AIDS Foundation. 2002 (http://www.

remedios.com.ph/fhtml/hivstat_articles_par.htm, accessed 23 February 2007).

Reproductive Health Outlook. Impact of gender role expectations on men's health. Seattle, PATH Reproductive Health Outlook, 2006 (www.rho.org/html/menrh_keyissues.htm, accessed 23 February 2007).

Rivers K., Aggleton P. *Adolescent sexuality, gender and the HIV epidemic.* New York, United Nations Development Programme, 1999.

Rothenberg K.H., Paskey S.J. The risk of domestic violence and women with HIV infection: implications for partner notification, public policy, and the law. *American Journal of Public Health,* 1995, 85(11):1569–1576.

Ruxin J., Binagwaho A., Wilson P.A. *Combating AIDS in the developing world.* New York, UN Millennium Project, Working Group on HIV/AIDS, 2005.

Safman R.M. Assessing the impact of orphanhood on Thai children affected by AIDS and their caregivers. *AIDS Care*, 2004, 16(1):11–19.

Scalway T. Young men and HIV-culture, poverty, and sexual *risk. Panos Report 41.* London, Panos Institute, 2001.

Schmader K.E. *et al.* HIV therapy works for older people too. *American Geriatrics Association*, 2002, 50:605–607.

Secretariat of the Pacific Community, the United Nations, UN/CROP MDG Working Group and United Nations. *The Pacific islands regional MDG report 2004.* Noumea, Secretariat of the Pacific Community, 2004.

Sodeco Social Development Consultants. *How to invest for future generations – guidelines for integrating HIV/AIDS in the development cooperation.* Stockholm, Swedish International Development Agency, 2002.

Sopheap H. *et al.* Rural sex work in Cambodia: work characteristics, risk behaviours, HIV, and syphilis. *Sexually Transmitted Infections,* 2003, 79:e2.

Soucat A., Yazbeck A. *Rapid guidelines for integrating health, nutrition and population issues in interim poverty reduction strategy papers of low-income countries.* Washington, D.C., World Bank, 2000 (http://www.worldbank.org/poverty/strategies/chapters/health/hnpguide.pdf, accessed 26 February 2007)

Sowell R. *et al.* Experiences of violence in HIV seropositive women in the south-eastern United States of America. *Journal of Advanced Nursing,* 1999, 30(3):606–615.

Steinberg M. *et al.* Hitting home. *How households cope with the impact of the HIV/AIDS epidemic: A survey of households affected by HIV/AIDS in South Africa.* Washington D.C., Henry J. Kaiser Family Foundation, 2002 (http://www.kff.org/southafrica/upload/Hitting-Home-How-Households-Cope-with-the-Impact-of-the-HIV-AIDS-Epidemic-Report.pdf, accessed 26 February 2007).

Sterling TR *et al.* Initial plasma HIV-1 RNA levels and progression to AIDS in women and men. *New England Journal of Medicine,* 2001, 344(10): 720-5.

Tallis V. *Gender and HIV/AIDS: Overview report.* Brighton, Institute of Development Studies, 2002 (http://www.bridge.ids.ac.uk/reports/cep-hiv-report.pdf, accessed 22 February 2007).

Tanner M., Vlassof C. Treatment-seeking behaviour for malaria: a typology based on endemicity and gender. *Social Science and Medicine,* 1998, 46(4-5):523–532.

Thang D.B. *et al*. Cross-sectional study of sexual behaviour and knowledge about HIV among urban, rural, and minority residents in Viet Nam. *Bulletin of the World Health Organization*, 2001, 79:15–21.

Thiede M. *et al*. South Africa: Who goes to the public sector for voluntary HIV/AIDS counselling and testing. HNP Discussion Paper Reaching the Poor Paper No. 6. Washington D.C., World Bank, 2004 (http://siteresources.worldbank.org/HEALTHNUTRITIONANDPOPULATION/Resources/281627-1095698140167/RPP6SAfrica.pdf, accessed 23 February 2007).

Timberlake S. *Men having sex with men and human rights: the UNAIDS perspective.* Paper presented at the ILGA World Conference Pre-Conference: MSM and Gay Men's Health. Geneva, UNAIDS, 2006.

Tran T.M. *et al*. HIV prevalence and factors associated with HIV infection among male injecting drug users under 30: a cross-sectional study in Long An, Vietnam. *BMC Public Health*. 2006, 6:248.

United Nations Population Fund. Enlisting men in HIV/AIDS prevention. Summarized from the report *Partners for change: enlisting men in HIV/AIDS prevention*. New York, UNFPA, 2000.

United Nations Population Fund. Prevention of HIV infection in pregnant women. HIV prevention now: Programme brief No. 2. New York, UNFPA, 2001 (http://www.unfpa.org/hiv/prevention/index.htm, accessed 23 February 2007).

United Nations Population Fund. Addressing gender perspectives in HIV prevention. HIV prevention now. Programme brief No. 4. New York, UNFPA, 2002 (http://www.unfpa.org/hiv/prevention/index.htm, accessed 23 February 2007).

United Nations Population Fund. *Culture matters. Working with communities and faith-based organizations: Case studies from country programmes*. New York, UNFPA, 2004.

United Nations Population Fund and World Health Organization Regional Office for the Western Pacific. *Meeting Report. Joint UNFPA/WHO Meeting on 100% Condom Use Programme, Manila, 3-6 October 2006*. Manila, UNFPA and WHO Regional Office for the Western Pacific, 2006.

United Nations. *HIV/AIDS and human rights: international guidelines*. New York and Geneva, Office of the United Nations High Commission for Human Rights and Joint United Nations Programme on HIV/AIDS, 1998.

United Nations Children's Fund. *HIV/AIDS: a top priority in coming years*. New York, UNICEF, 2001.

United Nations Children's Fund. Facts for life. New York, UNICEF, 2002a (www.unicef.org/ffl, accessed 23 February 2007).

United Nations Children's Fund. *The state of the world's children 2003*. New York, UNICEF, 2002b.

United Nations Children's Fund. *Children on the brink 2004. A joint report of new orphan estimates and a framework for action*. New York, UNICEF, Joint United Nations Programme on HIV/AIDS and United States Agency for International Development, 2004.

United Nations Children's Fund. *The state of the world's children 2005: childhood under threat*. New York, UNICEF, 2005.

United Nations Children's Fund. *The state of the world's children 2007. Women and children: the double dividend of gender equality*. New York, UNICEF, 2007 (http://www.unicef.org/sowc07/docs/sowc07.pdf, accessed 23 February 2007).

United Nations Children's Fund, Joint United Nations Programme on HIV/AIDS, World Health Organization. *Young people and HIV/AIDS: opportunity in crisis*. New York and Geneva, UNICEF, UNAIDS and WHO, 2002 (http://www.hivpolicy.org/Library/HPP000256.pdf, accessed 20 December 2007).

United Nations Country Team in China. *Millennium Development Goals: China's progress: an assessment by the UN Country Team in China*. Beijing, United Nations, 2004.

United Nations Country Team in Viet Nam. *Millennium Development Goals and Viet Nam's Socioeconomic Development Plan 2006-2010*. Ha Noi, United Nations, 2005.

United Nations Country Team in Viet Nam. *Millennium Development Goals: closing the Millennium gaps* (MDG Progress Report 2003). Ha Noi, United Nations, 2003 (http://www.un.org.vn/undocs/mdg03/mdg03e.pdf).

United Nations Development Fund for Women. *Transforming the national AIDS response: Gender equality, women's rights and the "Three Ones"*. New York, UNIFEM, 2008.

United Nations Development Programme. *Human development report 1995: gender and human development*. New York, Oxford University Press, 1995.

United Nations Development Programme. *National human development report Lao PDR 2001: advancing rural development*. Vientiane, UNDP, 2001.

United Nations Development Programme. *Transformation across borders addressing HIV/AIDS in the Asia Pacific Region: the answer lies within*. New York, UNDP, 2004 (http://www.undp.org/hiv/docs/regional_reps/asia_pacific_regional_report.pdf, accessed 23 February 2007).

United Nations Development Programme, South East Asia HIV and Development Programme. *African-Asian agriculture against AIDS*. Consultation on Agriculture, Development and HIV-vulnerability Reduction, 11–13 December 2002, Bangkok, Thailand. UNDP and Food and Agricultural Organization, 2004.

United Nations General Assembly. *Declaration of Commitment on HIV/AIDS: five years later. Report of the Secretary-General. Sixtieth session Agenda item 45*. New York, United Nations General Assembly, 2006 (http://data.unaids.org/pub/Report/2006/20060324_SGReport_GA_A60737_en.pdf, accessed 1 December 2006).

Urbang S. *Statement to UNGASS first informal consultative meeting*. New York, UNIFEM, 2001.

United States Centers for Disease Control and Prevention. HIV/AIDS among U.S. women: minority and young women at continuing risk. New York, Body Health Resources Corporation, 2001 (http://www.thebody.com/cdc/minority_women.html, accessed 23 February 2007).

United States Centers for Disease Control and Prevention. Human Immunodeficiency Virus Type 2. Washington, CDC, 1998 (http://www.cdc.gov/hiv/resources/factsheets/hiv2.htm, accessed 23 February 2007).

Van der Straten A. et al. Sexual coercion, physical violence, and HIV infection among women in steady relationships in Kigali, Rwanda. *AIDS and Behavior*, 1998, 2(1):61–73.

Van Rossem R., Meekers D. An evaluation of the effectiveness of targeted social marketing to promote adolescent and young adult reproductive health in Cameroon. *AIDS Education and Prevention*, 2000, 12.

Wagstaff A. Poverty and health sector inequalities. Bulletin of the World Health Organization, 2002, 80 (2):97–105 (www.who.int/bulletin/pdf/2002/bul-2-E-2002/80(2)97-105.pdf, accessed 26 February 2007).

Walford V. *Health in poverty reduction strategy papers (PRSPs): an introduction and early experience.* Brighton, Department for International Development Health Systems Resources Centre, 2001.

Walford V. *Cambodia: country health briefing paper.* London, Department for International Development, 2000.

Warwick I. *et al.,* Household and community responses to AIDS in developing countries. *Critical Public Health,* 1998, 84:291–310.

Wellings K. *et al.* Sexual behaviour in context: a global perspective. *The Lancet,* 2006, 368:1706–1728.

Wong M.L. *et al.* Social and behavioural factors associated with condom use among direct sex workers in Siem Reap, Cambodia. *Sexually Transmitted Infections,* 2003, 79:163–165.

Wood K. *et al. HIV prevention with especially vulnerable young people: case studies of success and innovation.* Geneva, World Health Organization and Department for International Development, 2006.

World Bank and International Monetary Fund. *Poverty reduction strategy programmes – progress in implementation.* Washington, D.C., World Bank and IMF, 2001.

World Bank. Confronting AIDS: public priorities in a global epidemic. Oxford, Oxford University Press, 1997 (http://www.worldbank.org/aidsecon/confront/, accessed 3 March 2007).

World Bank. *World development report 2004: making services work for poor people.* New York, Oxford University Press, 2003.

World Bank. *Development and poverty reduction. Looking back, looking ahead.* Speech by James D.Wolfensohn, François Bourguignon at the 2004 annual meeting of the World Bank and International Monetary Fund.*,* October 2004, Washington, D.C., World Bank, 2004.

World Bank. *World development indicators.* Washington, D.C., World Bank, 2006 (web.worldbank.org/WBSITE/EXTERNAL/DATASTATISTICS/0,,contentMDK:20421402~pagePK:64133150~piPK:64133175~theSitePK:239419,00.html, accessed 23 February 2007).

World Bank. *Millennium Development Goals.* Washington, D.C., World Bank, 2007 (http://ddp-ext.worldbank.org/ext/GMIS/home.do?siteId=2, accessed 23 February 2007).

World Bank. *Gender and HIV fact sheet: HIV/AIDS, gender and poverty.* Washington D.C., World Bank, n.d. a. (http://siteresources.worldbank.org/INTEAPREGTOPHIVAIDS/Resources/hivaidsgenderandpoverty_en_pdf.pdf, accessed 23 February 2007).

World Bank. *Gender and HIV fact sheet: rural HIV/AIDS.* Washington D.C., World Bank, n.d. b. (http://siteresources.worldbank.org/INTEAPREGTOPHIVAIDS/Resources/ruralhivaids_en_pdf.pdf, accessed 23 February 2007).

World Health Organization. *Women and AIDS: agenda for action.* Geneva, WHO, 1994.

World Health Organization. *The World Health Report 2000: health systems: improving performance.* Geneva, WHO, 2000a.

World Health Organization. *Fact sheets on HIV/AIDS for nurses and midwives* (WHO/EIP/OSD/2000.5). Geneva, WHO, 2000b.

World Health Organization. *Voluntary counselling and testing for HIV infection in antenatal care: practical considerations for implementation.* Geneva, WHO, 2000c.

World Health Organization. *Our health: health needs of women and girls affected by violence in Rwanda.* Geneva, WHO, 2000d.

World Health Organization. *Community home based care: family care giving for family members with HIV/AIDS and other chronic illnesses: a Botswana case study.* Geneva WHO, 2000e.

World Health Organization. *Health: a precious asset.* Geneva, WHO, 2000f (http://whqlibdoc.who.int/hq/2000/WHO_HSD_HID_00.1.pdf, accessed 26 February 2007).

World Health Organization. *Transforming health systems: gender and rights in reproductive health: a training curriculum for health programme managers.* Geneva, WHO, 2001a.

World Health Organization. *Investing in health: a summary of the findings of the Commission on Macroeconomics and Health.* Geneva, WHO, 2001b.

World Health Organization. *25 questions and answers on health and human rights.* Health and Human Rights Publication Series, Issue 1. Geneva, WHO, 2002a.

World Health Organization. *Gender and tuberculosis.* Geneva, WHO, 2002b. (http://www.who.int/gender/documents/en/TB.factsheet.pdf, accessed 27 February 2007).

World Health Organization. *Gender and HIV/AIDS.* Geneva, WHO, 2003a (http://www.who.int/gender/documents/en/Gender_factsheet.pdf, accessed 27 February 2007).

World Health Organization. *Integrating gender into HIV/AIDS programmes: a review paper.* Geneva, WHO, 2003b.

World Health Organization. *Emergency scale-up of antiretroviral therapy in resource limited settings: technical and operational recommendations to achieve 3 by 5.* Report of the WHO/UNAIDS International Consensus Meeting on Technical and Operational Recommendations for Emergency Scaling-Up of Antiretroviral Therapy in Resource-Limited Settings, 18–21 November 2003, Lusaka, Zambia. Geneva, WHO, 2003c.

World Health Organization. *Scaling up antiretroviral therapy in resource limited settings. Treatment guidelines for a public health approach.* Geneva, WHO, 2003d.

World Health Organization. *Integrating gender into HIV/AIDS programmes: a review paper.* Geneva, WHO, 2003e.

World Health Organization. *Guidance on ethics and equitable access to HIV treatment and care.* Geneva, WHO, 2004a.

World Health Organization. *The World Health Report 2004: changing history.* Geneva, WHO, 2004b.

World Health Organization. *TB/HIV: a clinical manual. Second edition.* Geneva, WHO, 2004c.

World Health Organization. *Ensuring equity between men and women in scaling up access to ART* (unpublished). Geneva, WHO, 2004d.

World Health Organization. *Interim patient monitoring guidelines for HIV care and ART.* Geneva, WHO, 2004e.

World Health Organization. *Standards for quality HIV care: a tool for quality assessment, improvement, and accreditation.* Geneva, WHO, 2004f.

World Health Organization. *Rapid HIV tests: guidelines for use in HIV testing and counseling services in resource-constrained settings.* Geneva, WHO, 2004g.

World Health Organization. *Human capacity-building plan for scaling up HIV/AIDS treatment.* Geneva, WHO, 2004h.

World Health Organization. *PRSPs, their significance for health: second synthesis report.* Geneva, WHO, 2004i.

World Health Organization. *Violence against women and HIV/AIDS: critical intersections. Intimate partner violence and HIV/AIDS.* Information Bulletin Series, Number 1. WHO and Global Coalition on Women and AIDS, 2004j (http://www.who.int/entity/gender/violence/en/vawinformationbrief.pdf, accessed 2007).

World Health Organization. *Violence against women and HIV/AIDS: critical intersections. Sexual violence in conflict settings and the risk of HIV.* Information Bulletin Series, Number 2. Geneva, WHO and Global Coalition on Women and AIDS, 2004k (http://www.who.int/entity/gender/en/infobulletinconflict.pdf, accessed 20 February 2007).

World Health Organization. *Violence against women and HIV/AIDS: information sheet.* Geneva, WHO and Global Coalition on Women and AIDS, 2004l (http://www.who.int/entity/gender/en/infosheetvawandhiv.pdf, accessed 20 February 2007).

World Health Organization. *Evidence for action on HIV/AIDS and injecting drug use. Policy brief: reduction of HIV transmission in prisons.* Geneva, WHO, 2004m (http://www.who.int/entity/hiv/pub/advocacy/en/transmissionprisonen.pdf, accessed 23 February 2007).

World Health Organization. *Integrating equity into health information systems.* Geneva, WHO, 2005a (http://www.who.int/healthmetrics/library/issue_3_05apr.doc, accessed 19 May 2005).

World Health Organization. *WHO multi-country study on women's health and domestic violence against women: initial results on prevalence, health outcomes and women's responses.* Geneva, WHO, 2005b (http://www.who.int/gender/violence/who_multicountry_study/en/index.html, accessed 3 March 2007).

World Health Organization. *The practice of charging user fees at point of service delivery for HIV/AIDS treatment and care.* Geneva, WHO, 2005c (http://www.who.int/entity/hiv/pub/advocacy/promotingfreeaccess.pdf, accessed 23 February 2007).

World Health Organization. *Antiretroviral drugs for treating pregnant women and preventing HIV infection in infants in resource-limited settings: towards universal access: recommendations for a public health approach, 2006 version.* Geneva, WHO, 2006a.

World Health Organization. *Scaling up HIV/AIDS prevention, treatment and care: a report on WHO's support to countries in implementing the "3 x 5" initiative 2005-2005.* Geneva, WHO, 2006b.

World Health Organization. *WHO Case definitions for HIV for surveillance and revised clinical staging and immunological classification.* Geneva, WHO, 2006c.

World Health Organization. *Towards universal access by 2010: How WHO is working with countries to scale-up HIV prevention, treatment and support.* Geneva, WHO, 2006d.

World Health Organization and Joint United Nations Programme on HIV/AIDS. *Accelerating access: summary of status for 4th meeting of contact group*. Geneva, WHO/UNAIDS Secretariat, 2002.

World Health Organization and Joint United Nations Programme on HIV/AIDS. *Fact sheet: progress in scaling up access to HIV treatment in low and middle-income countries, June 2006*. Geneva, WHO and UNAIDS, 2006.

World Health Organization and Joint United Nations Programme on HIV/AIDS. *UNAIDS/WHO policy statement on HIV testing*. Geneva, WHO and UNAIDS, 2004a.

World Health Organization and Joint United Nations Programme on HIV/AIDS. *Ensuring equitable access to antiretroviral treatment for women. WHO/UNAIDS Policy Statement*. Geneva, WHO, 2004b.

World Health Organization and World Bank. *Dying for change: poor people's experience of health and ill health*. Geneva, WHO, 2001.

World Health Organization Regional Office for the Western Pacific. *HIV/AIDS care and treatment: guide for implementation*. Manila, WHO Regional Office for the Western Pacific, 2004a.

World Health Organization Regional Office for the Western Pacific, Ministry of Health Republic of Kiribati, University of New South Wales, Australia. *Prevalence survey of sexually transmitted infections among seafarers and their women attending antenatal clinics in Kiribati*. Manila, WHO Regional Office for the Western Pacific, 2004b.

World Health Organization Regional Office for the Western Pacific. *HIV/AIDS in Asia and the Pacific Region 2003*. Manila, WHO Regional Office for the Western Pacific, 2004c (http://www.wpro.who.int/NR/rdonlyres/11ED3283-9821-43BE-9B73-B3444A3DADE6/0/HIV_AIDS_Asia_Pacific_Region2003.pdf, accessed 23 February 2007).

World Health Organization Regional Office for the Western Pacific. *Responding to questions about the 100% condom use programme: An aid for programme staff*. Manila, WHO Regional Office for the Western Pacific, 2004d.

World Health Organization Regional Office for the Western Pacific. *Participant manual: course 1A and 2A basic ART: HIV/AIDS clinical management for doctors, nurses and allied health workers at district/intermediate level*. Manila, WHO Regional Office for the Western Pacific, 2005a.

World Health Organization Regional Office for the Western Pacific. *Facilitator guide: course 1A and 2A basic ART: HIV/AIDS clinical management for doctors, nurses and allied health workers at district/intermediate level*. Manila, WHO Regional Office for the Western Pacific, 2005b.

World Health Organization Regional Office for the Western Pacific. *Meeting of Ministers of Health for the Pacific Island Countries Report, 14–17 March 2005, Apia, Samoa*. Manila, WHO Regional Office for the Western Pacific, 2005c.

World Health Organization Regional Office for the Western Pacific. *Report on UNAIDS/WHO Consultation on progress in prevention and care in the context of the "3 by 5 Initiative" and the perspective of universal access in the Western Pacific Region, 12-16 December 2005, Manila, Philippines*. WHO Regional Office for the Western Pacific, 2005d.

World Health Organization Regional Office for the Western Pacific. *Sexual and reproductive health of adolescents and youth in Cambodia: a review of literature and projects 1995-2003*. Manila, WHO Regional Office for the Western Pacific, 2005e.

World Health Organization Regional Office for the Western Pacific. HIV infection and surveillance. Manila, WHO Regional Office for the Western Pacific, 2005f (http://www.wpro.who.int/health_topics/hiv_infections/general_info.htm, accessed 23 February 2007).

World Health Organization Regional Office for the Western Pacific. The regional context. Manila, World Health Organization Regional Office for the Western Pacific, 2005g (http://www.wpro.who.int/sites/hsi/universal_access/regional_context.htm, accessed 23 February 2007).

World Health Organization Regional Office for the Western Pacific. Antiretroviral Therapy: 3 by 5 Initiative. Manila, World Health Organization Regional Office for the Western Pacific, 2005h (http://www.wpro.who.int/sites/hsi/universal_access/regional_context.htm, accessed 23 February 2007).

World Health Organization Regional Office for the Western Pacific. *Second generation surveillance surveys of HIV, other STIs and risk behaviours in six Pacific island countries.* Manila, WHO Regional Office for the Western Pacific, 2006.

World Health Organization Regional Office for the Western Pacific. *100% Condom Use Programme: experience from China (2001-2004): lessons learnt…future challenges.* Manila, WHO Regional Office for the Western Pacific, n.d.

Wyatt G.E. *et al.* Does a history of trauma contribute to HIV risk for women of color? Implications for prevention and policy. *American Journal of Public Health*, 2002, 92(4):660–665.

Xiao Y. *et al.* Expansion of HIV/AIDS in China: lessons from Yunnan Province. *Social Science and Medicine*, 2007,64:665–675.

Xiaoming L. *et al.* HIV/AIDS knowledge and the implications for health promotion programs among Chinese college students: geographic, gender and age differences. *Health Promotion International*, 2004, 19(3):345–356.

Xu K. *et al.* Household catastrophic health expenditure: a multicountry analysis. *The Lancet*, 2003, 362:111–117.

Yamey G., Rankin W.W. AIDS and global justice. *British Medical Journal*, 2002, 7331:181–182.

Yang H. *et al.* Living environment and schooling of children with HIV-infected parents in southwest China. *AIDS Care*, 2006, 18(7):647–655.

Yin L. *et al.* Continued spread of HIV among injecting drug users in southern Sichuan Province, China. *Harm Reduction Journal*, 2007, 4(6): doi:10.1186/1477-7517-4-6.

ENDNOTES

1. World Bank 2004.
2. United Nations Development Programme 1995.
3. Joint United Nations Programme on HIV/AIDS 2007g.
4. World Health Organization 2000a.
5. Bloom, River Path Associates, Sevilla 2002.
6. Medical Foundation for AIDS and Sexual Health 2003.
7. *Ibid*.
8. U.S. Centers for Disease Control and Prevention 1998.
9. World Health Organization 2000b.
10. World Health Organization 2006c.
11. *Ibid*.
12. *Ibid*.
13. Joint United Nations Programme on HIV/AIDS 2007g.
14. *Ibid*.
15. World Health Organization 2004b.
16. Joint United Nations Programme on HIV/AIDS 2006e.
17. Joint United Nations Programme on HIV/AIDS 2006a.
18. Joint United Nations Programme on HIV/AIDS 2006e.
19. Joint United Nations Programme on HIV/AIDS 2007g.
20. World Health Organization 2004b.
21. *Ibid*.
22. Joint United Nations Programme on HIV/AIDS 2007g.
23. *Ibid*.
24. *Ibid*.
25. *Ibid*.
26. Joint United Nations Programme on HIV/AIDS 2006e.
27. Joint United Nations Programme on HIV/AIDS 2007g.
28. *Ibid*.
29. Government of Papua New Guinea 2007.
30. Joint United Nations Programme on HIV/AIDS 2006a.
31. Joint United Nations Programme on HIV/AIDS 2007g.
32. World Health Organization Regional Office for the Western Pacific 2005f.
33. Monitoring the AIDS Pandemic Network 2001.
34. Joint United Nations Programme on HIV/AIDS 2006a.
35. Joint United Nations Programme on HIV/AIDS 2006e.
36. Joint United Nations Programme on HIV/AIDS 2006h.
37. *Ibid*.
38. World Health Organization Regional Office for the Western Pacific 2005f.
39. Joint United Nations Programme on HIV/AIDS 2006a.
40. Adeyi *et al.* 2001.
41. Joint United Nations Programme on HIV/AIDS 1999q.
42. Joint United Nations Programme on HIV/AIDS 2001a.
43. For more information on how poverty is conceptualized and measured, please refer to the foundational module on health and poverty in this series.
44. Lightfoot, Ryan 2001. The vulnerability of many developing countries in the Pacific to external shocks (including natural disasters and market failures) and their small resource base have led to their inclusion among Least Developed Countries. For more information on Least Developed Countries, Landlocked Developing Countries and Small Island Developing States, visit the website of the United Nations Office of the High Representative: (http://www.un.org/special-rep/ohrlls/ldc/default.htm).
45. Lampietti, Stalker 2000.
46. Adeyi *et al.* 2001.
47. *Ibid*.
48. Bloom, River Path Associates, Sevilla 2002; Beegle, De Weerdt, Dercon 2006.
49. Bloom, River Path Associates, Sevilla 2002.
50. *Ibid*. The study notes that this correlation remains significant even when African countries are removed from the analysis.
51. World Bank n.d a.
52. Bloom, River Path Associates, Sevilla 2002.
53. *Ibid*.
54. World Bank 1999. In: Beegle, De Weerdt, Dercon 2006.
55. De Walque 2006. In: Beegle, De Weerdt, Dercon 2006.
56. Bloom, River Path Associates, Sevilla 2002; Desbarats 2003; Masanjala 2007.
57. Parker 1998. In: Adeyi *et al.* 2001.
58. Cowan *et al.* 1994; Kreiger *et al.* 1990; McCoy *et al.* 1996. In: Adeyi *et al.* 2001.
59. Economies are divided according to 2005 GNI per capita, calculated using the World Bank Atlas method. The groups are: low income, US$ 875 or

less; lower middle income, US$ 876 – US$ 3465; upper middle income, US$ 3466 – US$ 10 725; and high income, US$ 10 726 or more. See World Bank, 2006.
60 China 2002. In: Desbarats 2003.
61 Action Aid 2005.
62 Adeyi *et al.* 2001.
63 Pitanyanon *et al.* 1997. In: Bloom, River Path Associates, Sevilla 2002.
64 Basu *et al.* 1997. In: Bloom, River Path Associates, Sevilla 2002.
65 Bloom *et al.* 1997. Socioeconomic dimensions of the HIV/AIDS epidemic in Sri Lanka. In: Bloom, River Path Associates, Sevilla 2002.
66 Bloom, River Path Associates, Sevilla 2002.
67 Walford 200l; Asian Development Bank 2002b; Asian Development Bank 2002d.
68 Lao People's Democratic Republic 2003.
69 World Bank n.d. b.
70 Qi 2002. In: World Bank n.d. b.
71 Passey *et al.* 1998.
72 Sopheab *et al.* 2003.
73 Xiaoming *et al.* 2004.
74 Gwatkin *et al.* 2007a.
75 Gwatkin *et al.* 2007b; Gwatkin *et al.* 2007c.
76 Gwatkin *et al.* 2007b.
77 Adeyi *et al.* 2001.
78 Bloom, River Path Associates, Sevilla 2002.
79 Van Landingham *et al.* 1997. In: Bloom, River Path Associates, Sevilla 2002.
80 Tran *et al.* 2006.
81 Bloom, River Path Associates, Sevilla 2002.
82 The International Community of Women Living with HIV/AIDS 2004.
83 Wong *et al.* 2003.
84 United Nations Population Fund 2003. In: Australian Agency for International Development and United Nations Development Programme 2005.
85 *Ibid.*
86 Wan and Zhang 2006. In: Joint United Nations Programme on HIV/AIDS 2006a.
87 Remedios AIDS Foundation 2002.
88 Joint United Nations Programme on HIV/AIDS 2002a.
89 Health Action Information Network 2005.
90 Shanghai Centres for Disease Control and Prevention 2004. In: He *et al.* 2006.
91 Huang 2002.
92 World Health Organization Regional Office for the Western Pacific, Ministry of Health Republic of Kiribati, University of New South Wales, Australia 2004.
93 David Lowe Consulting-Asia 2003.
94 United Nations Development Programme 2004.
95 Mateo *et al.* 2004.
96 Australian Agency for International Development and United Nations Development Programme 2005.
97 Joint United Nations Programme on HIV/AIDS 2006a.
98 Remedios AIDS Foundation 2002.
99 Korean UNAIDS Information Support Centre 2004.
100 Thant 1993. In: Bloom, Lyons (eds) 1993. In: Bloom, River Path Associates, Sevilla 2002.
101 Kaufman, Jing 2002.
102 Chenge *et al.* 1995. In: Xiao *et al.* 2007.
103 Lu *et al.* 2005. In: Xiao *et al.* 2007.
104 United States Centers for Disease Control and Prevention 2001.
105 Wyatt *et al.* 2002.
106 *Ibid.*
107 Asian Development Bank 2000. In: United Nations Development Programme 2001.
108 Health Action Information Network 2005.
109 United Nations Children's Fund 2002b.
110 Health Action Information Network 2005.
111 United Nations Country Team Viet Nam 2003.
112 United Nations Children's Fund 2007.
113 Rivers, Aggleton 1999.
114 United Nations Country Team Viet Nam 2005.
115 HelpAge International 2002.
116 Gwatkin *et al.* 2007c.
117 Passey *et al.* 1998.
118 *Ibid.*
119 Government of the Lao People's Democratic Republic and the United Nations 2004.
120 World Health Organization 2000e.
121 Gwatkin *et al.* 2007a.
122 Gwatkin *et al.* 2007b.
123 Ivers *et al.* 2005.
124 Health Action Information Network 2005.
125 Chalker *et al.* 2000.
126 Hesketh *et al.* 2005. In: UNAIDS 2006a.
127 World Health Organization, Department of Gender and Women's Health 2003.
128 Lau, Tsul 2005.
129 Schmader *et al.* 2002.
130 Wagstaff suggests that quality of care may be broadly defined as including services and amenities, as well as technical quality. Wagstaff 2002.
131 Ministry of Planning, Kingdom of Cambodia

131. 2001.
132. Government of Mongolia and United Nations Development Programme 2003.
133. McMurry 2004.
134. Organization for Economic Cooperation and Development and World Health Organization 2003.
135. Government of Mongolia and United Nations Development Programme 2003.
136. World Bank 2003.
137. World Health Organization and World Bank 2001.
138. Thiede *et al.* 2004.
139. Passey *et al.* 1998.
140. Dwyer 2004.
141. Chalke *et al.* 2000.
142. Lui, Hsiao. In: World Health Organization 2001b.
143. World Health Organization 2003d.
144. Hardon *et al.* 2006.
145. Kumarasamy *et al.* 2005.
146. Adeyi *et al.* 2001.
147. Masanjala 2007.
148. World Health Organization 2001b.
149. *Ibid.*
150. Joint United Nations Programme on HIV/AIDS 2000e.
151. Adeyi *et al.* 2001.
152. World Health Organization 2000a.
153. Bloom, River Path Associates, Sevilla 2002.
154. Viravaidya *et al.* 1992. In: Australian Agency for International Development and United Nations Development Programme 2005; and Bloom *et al.* 2002. In: Australian Agency for International Development and United Nations Development Programme 2005.
155. Adeyi *et al* 2001.
156. World Health Organization 2004c.
157. United Nations Development Programme 2003. In: Action Aid 2005.
158. Knodel 2005.
159. Adeyi *et al.* 2001.
160. *Ibid.*
161. Steinberg *et al.* 2002.
162. Beegle, De Weerdt, Dercon. 2006.
163. Pitayanon *et al.* 1994. In: Australian Agency for International Development and United Nations Development Programme 2005.
164. Soucat, Yazbeck 2000.
165. Joint United Nations Programme on HIV/AIDS 1999. In: World Health Organization 2000f.
166. *HIV/AIDS and food security*. Ottawa, International Coalition on AIDS and Development, 2001.
167. United Nations Development Programme, South East Asia HIV and Development Programme 2004.
168. Joint United Nations Programme on HIV/AIDS 2000w.
169. Human Rights Watch 2006.
170. Hunter, Williamson 1996.
171. Yang *et al.* 2006.
172. United Nations Children's Fund 2002a.
173. Safman 2004.
174. Joint United Nations Programme on HIV/AIDS 2007d.
175. Population Division of the Department of Economic and Social Affairs of the United Nations Secretariat 2002, *World Population prospects: the 2000 revision*. In: United Nations Country Team Viet Nam 2005.
176. Id21 2002b.
177. Bonnel 2000.
178. *Ibid.*
179. World Health Organization 2004b.
180. Joint United Nations Programme on HIV/AIDS 2002a.
181. Tallis 2002.
182. Joint United Nations Programme on HIV/AIDS 1999c.
183. Joint United Nations Programme on HIV/AIDS 2007g.
184. Joint United Nations Programme on HIV/AIDS 2004b.
185. Joint United Nations Programme on HIV/AIDS 2001c.
186. United Nations Population Fund 2002.
187. Id21 2002a.
188. World Health Organization 2000d.
189. Joint United Nations Programme on HIV/AIDS 1997c.
190. World Health Organization 2000b.
191. United Nations Population Fund 2002.
192. Duvvury, Knoess 2005.
193. Adeyi *et al.* 2001.
194. Duvvury, Knoess 2005.
195. Cash, Anasuchatkul 1995.
196. United Nations Children's Fund 2002a.
197. United Nations Population Fund 2001.
198. Id21 2002d.
199. Joint United Nations Programme on HIV/AIDS 1998d.
200. Joint United Nations Programme on HIV/AIDS 2002a.
201. Joint United Nations Programme on HIV/AIDS 1997f.

202 World Health Organization 1994.
203 Tallis 2002.
204 Joint United Nations Programme on HIV/AIDS 1997c.
205 Tallis 2002.
206 Chesney, Smith 1999.
207 World Health Organization 2004j; World Health Organization 2005b.
208 World Health Organization 2004j.
209 Martin *et al.* 1999. In: World Health Organization 2004j.
210 World Health Organization 2005b.
211 World Health Organization 2000b.
212 Warwick *et al.*, 1998.
213 Esplen 2007.
214 Centre for Reproductive Rights 2005. In: Esplen 2007.
215 Aggleton, Warwick. 1999.
216 FWLD 2002. In: Paxton *et al.* 2004.
217 de Bruyn *et al.* 2002. In: Paxton *et al.* 2004.
218 Asia Pacific Network of People Living with HIV/AIDS 2004. In: Paxton *et al.* 2004.
219 World Health Organization 2004b.
220 Centre for HIV/AIDS Networking, University of KwaZulu-Natal 2005.
221 Sterling *et al.* 2001.
222 Napravnik *et al.* 2002.
223 Tallis 2002.
224 Ford, Koetsawang 1991.
225 World Health Organization Regional Office for the Western Pacific 2005e.
226 United Nations Population Fund 2004.
227 Centre for HIV/AIDS Networking, University of KwaZulu-Natal 2005.
228 Duvvury, Knoess 2005.
229 Joint United Nations Programme on HIV/AIDS 2000m.
230 United Nations Population Fund 2000.
231 Orubuloye, Caldwell, Caldwell 1993.
232 Joint United Nations Programme on HIV/AIDS 1999m.
233 World Health Organization 2000b.
234 Reproductive Health Outlook 2006.
235 Gordon, Sleightholme. n.d.
236 Joint United Nations Programme on HIV/AIDS 1997i.
237 Aggleton *et al.* 1996.
238 Engender Health 2006.
239 Mane 1997.
240 Joint United Nations Programme on HIV/AIDS 1998g.
241 World Health Organization 2004m.
242 Dolan *et al.* 2004
243 Human Rights Watch n.d.
244 Joint United Nations Programme on HIV/AIDS, 2007e.
245 Braveman, Gruskin 2003a.
246 World Health Organization 2001a.
247 Joint United Nations Programme on HIV/AIDS 2006e.
248 Joint United Nations Programme on HIV/AIDS 2006a.
249 *Ibid.*
250 United Nations Population Fund 2002.
251 World Health Organization 2002b.
252 MacNaughton 2004.
253 Jurgens, Cohen n.d.
254 General comment on the right to the highest attainable standard of health, article 12 ICESCR in WHO 2002a.
255 Tallis 2002.
256 Office of the United Nations High Commissioner for Human Rights 2000.
257 Joint United Nations Programme on HIV/AIDS 2001e.
258 United Nations 1998.
259 Joint United Nations Programme on HIV/AIDS 2002a.
260 World Health Organization 2005c.
261 Joint United Nations Programme on HIV/AIDS 2006f.
262 For more information on the Commission on Social Determinants of Health, please see: (http://www.who.int/social_determinants/en/).
263 Walford 2001.
264 Lao People's Democratic Republic 2003 and Joint United Nations Programme on HIV/AIDS, United Nations Development Programme, World Bank 2005.
265 Government of Mongolia 2003.
266 World Health Organization and Joint United Nations Programme on HIV/AIDS 2004b.
267 Joint United Nations Programme on HIV/AIDS 2007f.
268 Adeyi *et al.* 2001.
269 Joint United Nations Programme on HIV/AIDS 2006f.
270 World Health Organization and UNAIDS 2004b.
271 Gwatkin 2002.
272 World Bank 1997.
273 World Health Organization and Joint United Nations Programme on HIV/AIDS 2004b; World Health Organization 2003e.
274 World Health Organization Regional Office for

275. the Western Pacific 2005c.
275. Global Fund to Fight AIDS, Malaria and Tuberculosis 2006.
276. World Health Organization and Joint United Nations Programme on HIV/AIDS 2002.
277. World Health Organization 2006d.
278. Joint United Nations Programme on HIV/AIDS 1998f.
279. World Health Organization and UNAIDS 2004b.
280. Ibid.
281. World Health Organization 2003e.
282. For more detailed information, please see the resources listed in Section 6 (Tools and Resources).
283. World Health Organization Regional Office for the Western Pacific 2005h.
284. Joint United Nations Programme on HIV/AIDS 2006f.
285. It should be noted that the checklist addresses only the health services that relate to gender, poverty and HIV/AIDS within general health care practice.
286. World Health Organization Regional Office for the Western Pacific 2005g.
287. Id21 2002c.
288. United Nations Population Fund 2002.
289. Barker 1999.
290. Panos Institute 2001.
291. Scalway 2001.
292. Risky sexual relations are defined as those involving penetration and/or the risk of exposure to bodily fluids.
293. World Health Organization Regional Office for the Western Pacific 2004c.
294. United Nations Population Fund and World Health Organization Regional Office for the Western Pacific 2006.
295. World Health Organization Regional Office for the Western Pacific n.d.
296. World Health Organization Regional Office for the Western Pacific 2004c.
297. Ibid.
298. David Lowe Consulting-Asia 2003.
299. United Nations Population Fund and World Health Organization Regional Office for the Western Pacific 2006.
300. Joint United Nations Programme on HIV/AIDS 2006c.
301. Joint United Nations Programme on HIV/AIDS 2005.
302. Ibid.
303. Ibid.
304. Ibid.
305. Kamali *et al.* 2002.
306. World Health Organization 2006a.
307. Ibid.
308. Ibid.
309. Preble, Piwoz 2002.
310. Esplen 2007.
311. World Health Organization 2000c.
312. Rothenberg, Paskey 1995.
313. Joint United Nations Programme on HIV/AIDS 2000s.
314. DeCarlo 2000.
315. World Health Organization 2004g.
316. Joint United Nations Programme on HIV/AIDS 2007b.
317. Ibid.
318. World Health Organization and Joint United Nations Programme on HIV/AIDS 2006.
319. World Health Organization and Joint United Nations Programme on HIV/AIDS 2004.
320. Population Council 2001.
321. World Health Organization and Joint United Nations Programme on HIV/AIDS 2004.
322. Ibid.
323. Maman *et al.* 2003.
324. Ruxin, Binagwaho, Wilson 2005.
325. Although not a cure, ART increases the quality of life of people living with HIV/AIDS, in addition to easing the burden of care on families and health systems. ART reduces mortality by up to 90% and the risk of major opportunistic infections by 55%–80%, at least in the first years of treatment. Ruxin, Binagwaho, Wilson 2005.
326. World Health Organization Regional Office for the Western Pacific 2005g.
327. World Health Organization 2006b.
328. World Health Organization Regional Office for the Western Pacific 2005d.
329. World Health Organization 2004b.
330. Joint United Nations Programme on HIV/AIDS 2006a.
331. World Health Organization and Joint United Nations Programme on HIV/AIDS 2004b.
332. World Health Organization 2004b.
333. World Health Organization and Joint United Nations Programme on HIV/AIDS 2004b.
334. World Health Organization 2006d.
335. World Health Organization 2005c.
336. Hardon *et al.* 2006.
337. World Health Organization and Joint United Nations Programme on HIV/AIDS 2006.
338. World Health Organization and Joint United Nations Programme on HIV/AIDS 2004b.

339. Tanner, Vlassoff 1998.
340. Organization for Economic Cooperation and Development and World Health Organization 2003.
341. World Health Organization 2004f.
342. World Health Organization 2004h.
343. Joint United Nations Programme on HIV/AIDS 2006a.
344. International Labour Organization/World Health Organization 2005.
345. Paterson *et al.* 2000. In: Hardon *et al.* 2006.
346. *Ibid.*
347. Ruxin, Binagwaho, Wilson 2005.
348. *Ibid.*
349. World Health Organization 2005a.
350. *Ibid.*
351. World Health Organization 2004b.
352. Joint United Nations Programme on HIV/AIDS 1998h.